Also by

CHRYS CHRYSSANTHOU

* * * * *

CRIES AND WHISPERS
Anthology of Poems

THE SECRET MESSAGE OF THE ROOSTER
And Other Amazing Stories during the Nazi Occupation

HOW TO KEEP YOUNG
A prescription to Ageless Aging

LONGER YOUTH
&
BETTER MEMORY

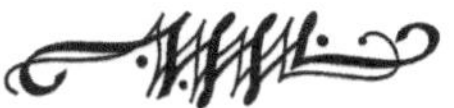

A PRESCRIPTION TO ACHIEVE
AGELESS AGING

CHRYS CHRYSSANTHOU

Ordering Information:

For orders and inquiries, please contact:
1-888-404-1388
www.goldtouchpress.com
book.orders@goldtouchpress.com

Printed in the United States of America

Praise for

CRIES AND WHISPER

"Some of the poems made me shiver and brought me close to tears ... His poems reveal the human condition, both the good and the awful, and encapsulate moments of sadness, quiet joy, love and humanity—the cries and whispers."

—Dr. E. Thomopoulos,
Managing Editor of "Books,"
The National Herald, (New York,NY)

"Milestone in Greek America ... poetry reflecting on nature's mysteries and gifts and life forces."

—*Greek America Magazine,* Chicago, Illinois

"One of the Best Collections of Poetry ... thought provoking and moving."

—Ali--Arizona Music Fun, (Phoenix, AZ)

THE SECRET MESSAGE OF THE ROOSTER

"The stories are incredible ... unique and highly entertaining ... about life, survival, free spirit, heroic acts and a desire for excitement."

—*Greek America Magazine,* (Chicago, IL)

Chryssanthou enthusiastically recounts his experiences with spirit, suspense and humanity.

Apolo-Apseind Book Review, (USA)

"The stories are at once poignant, exciting, humorous and riveting … a great storyteller."

Ali-Arizona Music Fun, (Phoenix, AZ)

HOW TO KEEP YOUNG

"Chryssanthou said How to Keep Young is unique because in addition to the important role of exercise in maintaining youth, it emphasizes the pivotal role of self –perception, mindset and certain behavioral activities."

Eleni Sakellis
The National Herald (New York, NY)

The prescription provides guidance to help adults of all ages maintain youthfulness and health both physically and mentally.

BBW Book News (USA)

Contents

PART 1
FOUNTAINS AND ELIXIRS OF YOUTH

PART 2
THE PRESCRIPTION FOR LONGER YOUTH

PART 3
THE PRESCRIPTION FOR A BETTER MEMORY

To my daughters, Depy and Elena.

Acknowledgments

What triggered the writing of this book was the exhortation that I experienced by several of my friends. Their arguments and their urging me to disseminate my thoughts and my advice on aging gave me incentive and purpose. I thank them for that.

A considerable part of my research and writing was done in a very unusual environment: in the huge and quiet library of *Queen Mary 2* during a two-week cruise to the Caribbean. I greatly appreciate the opportunity I was given to couple my intense and taxing intellectual work with the relaxation of a sea voyage.

The Internet too deserves an acknowledgment for the help it provided for my research.

I also I like to express my appreciation to Jo Ann Gambale for her counsel on legal matters and to Helen Daman for her editorial help. Helen went meticulously, line by line, through my drafts and made important remarks and valuable suggestions.

But above all, I am deeply grateful to my wonderful wife, Gabriele, for her support and encouragement and for graciously tolerating my frequent and lengthy periods of being incommunicado.

Prologue

At my 90th birthday celebration, many of my guests could not believe that I am that old. This was not surprising to me because very often, when I disclose my age, I encounter the same disbelief and amazement. This reaction, I believe, is elicited by my vibrant behavior and my vivacious mannerism and demeanor, rather than by my youngish appearance. Several people asked me how do I manage to keep young? What is my secret?

Having anticipated the bewilderment and the expected curiosity, I had decided, in lieu of giving the customary speech for the occasion, to do something unusual and unique.

To reveal my "secret"!

After I blew the candles of my huge birthday cake, I climbed on the stage, grabbed the microphone from the lectern and following some greetings and introductory remarks, I disclosed my secret to a surprised, spellbound audience. I revealed my

prescription for staying young and active. I revealed my "Elixir*
of Youth."

The response was overwhelming. At the end of the party, I
was surrounded by a lot of guests and inundated by comments
and questions. They wanted me to elaborate more and clarify
certain points. Many asked if I had copies of my speech or if it
had been recorded. No, there was no recording and no copies. I
had spoken extemporaneously. They urged me to make a DVD.

I considered their advice, and after some time of contemplation
I concluded that publicizing my prescription might help some
people improve their lives. But instead of recording a DVD I
decided to disseminate the information by writing a book.

This is how the book "How to Keep Young" was born.

Some of the older readers pointed out to me that one of the
undesirable effects of aging that frustrates them most, is the
memory lapses. They commented that, perhaps, the book would
have been better if it had addressed this issue, which is a key
concern of many people, particularly seniors.

Their remarks made sense and now, four years later, I revised
the book, added a new section on memory and how to improve
it and gave it a new title: *"Longer Youth &Better Memory."*

The book reveals how I have been keeping myself young.
How, being ninety-four years old, I am still able to go to the
gym everyday, run on the treadmill and lift weights, play tennis,
bicycle, swim, dance, and be very active academically, socially
and intellectually. Just having a good DNA, without following
my prescription, would not have been enough to afford me those
activities.

---

* Elixir refers to a wonder substance (potion) once believed to sustain
youth and prolong life; a magical cure.

My prescriptions, my Elixirs, are not a magic potion. Nor are they promising wonder drug. My prescriptions are primarily for behavioral precepts. They are a set of guidelines for specific actions and the adoption of a particular mentality.

The prescription for a longer youth does not claim to remove your wrinkles, although it may improve the condition of your skin and your expression and give you a youngish appearance. It will not give you a baby face, but it could give you a baby's zest for life.

The prescription for a better memory could help you avoid the handicap of forgetfulness and give you greater self-confidence and more freedom in mental functions.

Both prescriptions could give you greater vigor and vitality and a vibrant disposition. It could give you a happier, more productive and fulfilling life.

Chrys Chryssanthou, M.D.

Important Admonition

The information and advice in this book should not be construed as a claim or promise of any kind of benefits or a guarantee of any particular results.

The health measures advocated herein, including but not limited to diets, medical checkups, vaccinations, sleep, and exercises, may not be appropriate for some people and should not be implemented without prior medical consultation with a physician.

The author, the publisher, and their editors disclaim any responsibility or liability for any damages or losses resulting from any advice or recommendation given in this book.

Introduction

In a civilized society, it is natural and expected that the young will attract a lot of attention of its citizens and of its institutions. Education, entertainment, sports, advertising, fashion—they are all aimed and geared primarily to the new generations.

We admire the energy and vitality of the young, and we are captivated by their young look and by the allure of the fresh faces and the willowy bodies. But in the culture of our modern society, this attention and admiration has become an obsession. We are enthralled with youth and we dread old age because we are inundated with messages that old age is plagued with misery. This idolization of youth and the gloomy perception of aging reached a point of a certain stigma being attached to old age. This, in turn, led to consider seniors a burden on society. Women are particularly self-conscious and concerned with the effects of aging on their appearance, especially regarding wrinkles, graying hair, and sagging skin.

They try to find remedies in cosmetics, plastic surgery, and other medical interventions, often becoming victims of ineffective creams and lotions and dubious cosmetic procedures.

Also, as we grow older, we experience memory problems which some of us are trying, unsuccessfully, to remedy with wander pills and dubious extracts.

Most of us wish we could stay young forever, but we are not Adaline, as she was in the 2015 fantasy movie "The Age of Adaline" nor are we Dorian Grey, as he was in Oscar Wild's "Picture of Dorian Grey".

There is no magic bullet for perpetual youth as there is no magic way to achieve perpetual motion. We cannot achieve eternal youth, but we can hope to be able to achieve a more youthful aging.

Because of the dramatic increase in the aging population in the last part of the twentieth century, scientists, in many parts of the world tried to find ways to ameliorate old age. A lot of attention was paid to the so called "Successful Aging". This term, and the objective it represents, though not exactly the same as "Longer Youth and Better Memory," is close enough to have relevance to the subject of my prescriptions.

There have been numerous studies on successful aging which is a multidimensional concept that can be traced back to the 1950s. Two principal models-definitions of the term "successful aging" were proposed: biomedical and socio-psychological.

The biomedical models emphasize absence of disease and good physical and mental functioning as successful aging. The original work in the biomedical category was conducted by the MacArthur Foundation.*

---

*   The MacArthur Foundation, through grants and loans, provides support for programs that foster development of knowledge.

The socio-psychological models underscore life satisfaction, social functioning and participation, or psychological resources.[1] A group of investigators combined the two models and defined successful aging as absence or avoidance of disease and risk factors for disease, maintenance of physical and cognitive functioning, and active engagement with life (including maintenance of autonomy and social support).[2]

My prescriptions differ substantially from those models. There may be an overlap with some elements in "successful aging," but my prescription emphasizes the crucial influence that certain changes in attitude and psychological orientation may exert on aging.

We do not know what exactly causes aging.

There is a quagmire of competing theories. Gerontological research involving genetics, neurology, metabolism, biochemistry and physiology, is booming, but the holy grail of aging is still elusive. There are still misconceptions that are, at least partially, responsible for suffering the undesirable manifestations of aging. Most of us have been led to believe that cognitive decline is inevitable. Dementia and even Alzheimer's disease are hanging like the *Sword of Damocles**over our heads. We were also led to believe that our bodies decline, that life becomes less enjoyable and fulfilling and that generally we are going downhill.

We may accept those misconceptions as a fact of life, or we may abandon them and adopt a more optimistic attitude and a positive self-perception of aging.

How we perceive aging can actually influence how we age. With a positive perception and some adjustments in our

---

* The sword of Damocles, according to Greek mythology, is an allusion to an imminent and ever present peril and constant fear.

lifestyle, we may be able to prevent, attenuate, and even reverse the frailty of aging.

My book provides incentives, mental tools, and precepts for achieving this goal.

The instructions for each particular objective are given with the corresponding rationale, and, whenever appropriate and possible, with the scientific basis.

Once I made up my mind to write a book about my prescription for longer youth and better memory, I decided to broaden the topic and provide a historical review of myths and facts regarding "elixirs" and "fountains of youth". A brief digest of what our ancestors believed could give them eternal youth and a look at the state of the art of modern sciences regarding their quest for an elixir that would prevent, delay or even reverse the deterioration associated with old age.

This information will place my prescriptions in perspective and on a relevant background.

Our bodies are our gardens—our wills are our gardeners.

—WILLIAM SHAKESPEARE

Lack of activity destroys the good condition of every human being, while movement and methodical physical exercise save it and preserve it.

—PLATO

PART 1

Fountains And Elixirs Of Youth

Facts and Myths

One of the fundamental realities in the cosmos is the universal cycle of existence: Birth-Death-Birth-Death; Light-Darkness-Light. Stars are being born, and stars are dying. They are created, they shine, they radiate their young splendor, they mature, and eventually, they die. Light beacons at one time, black holes the next.

So does nature on our planet. It follows the cycle: spring, summer, fall, winter, and then spring again. New life in springtime. An orgy of colors, of fragrances, and the vibrant tweeting of the birds. Young buds and tender leaves on the trees and the green velvet of fresh grass on the ground. A feast of life in the summer. But then comes fall and winter. Naked branches, bare trees, and fallen dead leaves on the ground. Creation in the spring, demise in the winter.

The cycle of nature.

The cycle of existence.

Mankind became aware of this cycle from the very beginning. We are all conscious of the fact that we are unavoidably tethered to the cycle of existence: birth, youth, aging, death.

And while all of us have accepted and surrendered to the inescapable certainty of death, some of us have been challenging the inevitability of aging.

The creeping deterioration of mental capacity, the loss of vitality and sometimes of libido, made us fearful of getting old and led us to seek ways to avert the frailty of aging. Homer called old age loathsome, and Shakespeare characterized it as hideous winter.

The quest for a way to preserve youth has consumed mankind for thousands of years. Throughout the eons, people used a variety of methods in an attempt to fend off the ravages of the senior years. They searched for something they could do, drink, or eat that would give them eternal youth.

Looking back in history, we find gods and mortals in the same boat. The Greek gods of Mount Olympus, however, managed, as legend has it, to achieve eternal youth and immortality by eating ambrosia[*] and drinking nectar. The poor mortals, on the other hand, have been engaged in an endless quest for the holy grail of eternal youth. They tried magic potions and searched for miraculous waters in rivers and fountains that, they believed, would restore the body to its prime. Stories about wondrous drinks and mysterious places with magical waters were spread throughout the world and through many generations.

This is how the myths and the legends of fountains and elixirs of youth were generated and disseminated.

---

[*] Mythological food of ancient Greek deities, allegedly deriving from the horns of a magical goat, giving them strength and power, youth and immortality.

But the interest and quest for methods to prevent or reverse aging are not a monopoly of mythology. Even at present, we are seeking ways to preserve our youth.

We dread old age, and we are willing to try anything to achieve this elusive goal.

Cosmetics and medical interventions are used to give us a youthful face, and with pharmaceuticals and other chemical compounds, we are attempting to avert the cognitive failures and losses in capability that accompany old age.

With the progress in the biochemistry, physiology, and genetics of the aging process, scientists are trying to prevent, retard, and even reverse aging by pharmacological means or by genomic manipulations. Despite the exciting and encouraging results of some studies, however, production and availability of an effective and safe elixir of youth does not seem imminent.

Before we get a glimpse at the state-of-the-art modern elixirs and fountains of youth, let us have a look at the history of those panaceas.[*]

---

[*]   A word derived from the Greek referring to something that is supposed to cure all diseases and solve every problem.

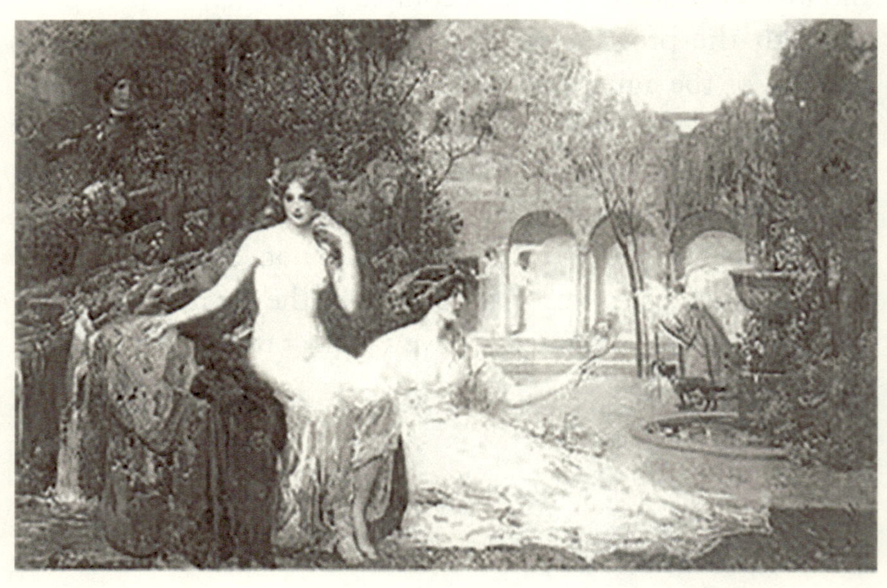

A painting by the Austrian artist Eduard Veith depicting a legendary fountain of youth.

Fountains of Youth

Fountains of youth are mythical fountains with mystical rejuvenating properties and ability to restore youth of anyone who drinks or bathes in their waters. They originated from mythical tales and folklore that have been recounted across the globe for many centuries.

One of the earliest, if not the first, reference to a fountain of youth takes us back to fifth century BC, when the Greek historian Herodotus wrote of a fountain in the land of Macrobians (an area in modern-day Somalia), which gave the people of the region exceptionally long life spans. When they washed with the water of the fountain, *they found their flesh all glossy and sleek as if they had bathed in oil and a scent came from the spring like that of violets.*[3]

Another story of a quest for eternal youth in the ancient world concerns the alleged attempts of Alexander the Great to find the fountain of youth.

According to the Eastern versions of the *Alexander Romance*, the king of the Macedonians crossed a mythical land covered in eternal night (the "Land of Darkness") to get to the river that could reverse aging.

This legend sounds somewhat unrealistic because at the time of his expeditions, Alexander was too young to worry about aging, unless he was seeking to preserve his vigor and youth in order to be able to complete his conquests and enjoy the spoils for a long, long time.

In the ensuing centuries, many myths and legends circulated, describing fountains and rivers with the magical power of rejuvenation.

A mythical king in the Orient, known as Prester John, who reigned during the twelfth century AD, ruled a land that, according to the legend, had a river of gold and a fountain of youth.

Another fountain of youth was supposed to be located at the foot of a mountain outside Polombe (modern Kollan) in India.[4]

In Japan, stories of hot springs that can restore youth are still circulating to this day.

In the fifth century AD, the newly discovered world of the Americas became a fertile ground for myths and fantasies of miraculous springs and fountains of youth.

Legend has it that the Caribbean Islanders, the Arawaks, spoke of Bimini, a mythical land located on Boinca, an island in the Gulf of Honduras, that, allegedly, had a fountain of youth. Taino Indians of the Caribbean also spoke of a magic fountain and a rejuvenating river somewhere north of Cuba.

The Italian geographer Pietro Martire d'Anghiera wrote,

> *Among the islands of the north side of Hispaniola, about 325 leagues distant, as said by those who have searched for it, is a continual spring of flowing water of such marvelous virtue that the water thereof being drunk, perhaps with some diet, maketh old men young again.*

The most persistent, however, and perhaps the best-known story of a search for the fountain of youth is the one involving the Spanish explorer Juan Ponce de Leon in sixteenth century AD. According to sketchy and undocumented information, King Ferdinand of Spain gave Ponce de Leon permission to mount an expedition to the Caribbean Islands to find the city of gold. But one historian suggested a different motive. He wrote that King Ferdinand, who had recently married a woman thirty-five years his junior, asked Ponce de Leon to explore the Caribbean but with the task of keeping an eye for the fountain of youth!

According to the chief historian of the Indies, in AD 1596, Ponce de Leon sent out a ship to find the island of Bimini, which the Indians had alleged was the site of a fountain that turned old men into boys! The ship came back and reported that Bimini had been found but not the fountain. Ponce de Leon left Puerto Rico, of which he was the governor in AD 1513, to get to the uncharted island of Bimini, but instead, he eventually landed in Florida, where he staked a claim for the Spanish Crown.

There are various theories regarding the incentives that stimulated Ponce de Leon's expeditions. Some writers alleged that his motivation was political: a hope for a profitable governorship. He was also very ambitious, and perhaps he wanted to gain a spot in the annals of history. Others have suggested it was his insatiable thirst for youth and eternity that drove him to the search for the fountain of youth.[5] There are even those who believed that Ponce de Leon sought the fountain of youth in a misguided attempt to cure his impotence.

Regardless of his motivation, the fact remains that most accounts of that period maintained that the main goal of Ponce de Leon was to discover the fountain of youth. Legend holds that during his Florida expedition, he and a few of his trusted men would go off unofficially in search of the elusive fountain.

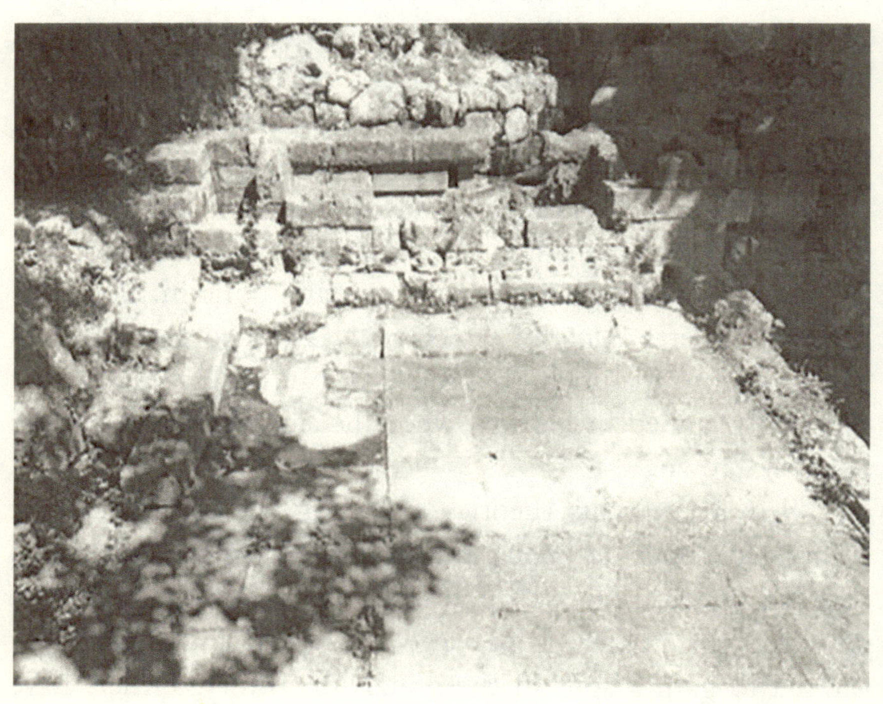

Ancient Greeks bathed here to gain eternal youth.

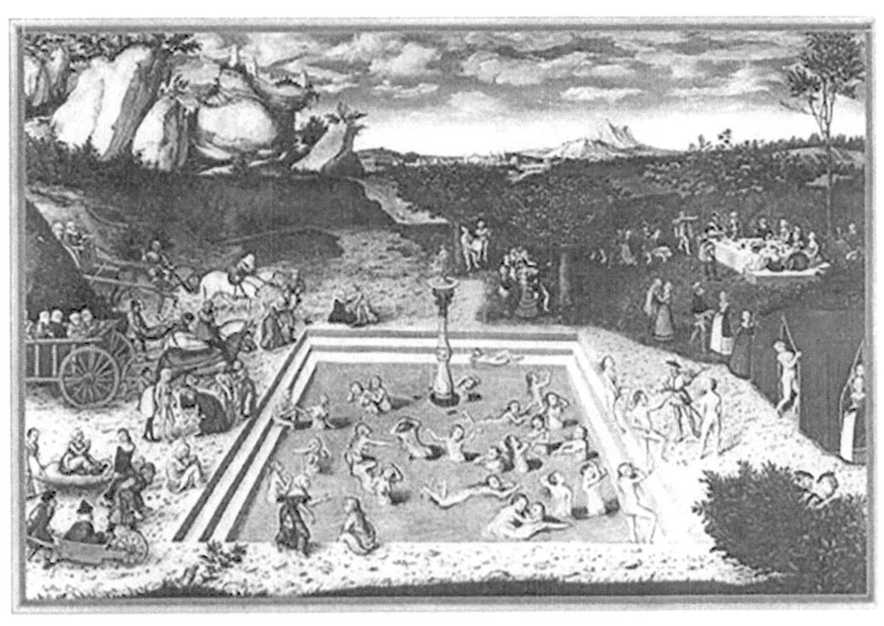

An AD 1546 painting of Lucas Cranach the Elder showing people bathing in a fountain of youth.

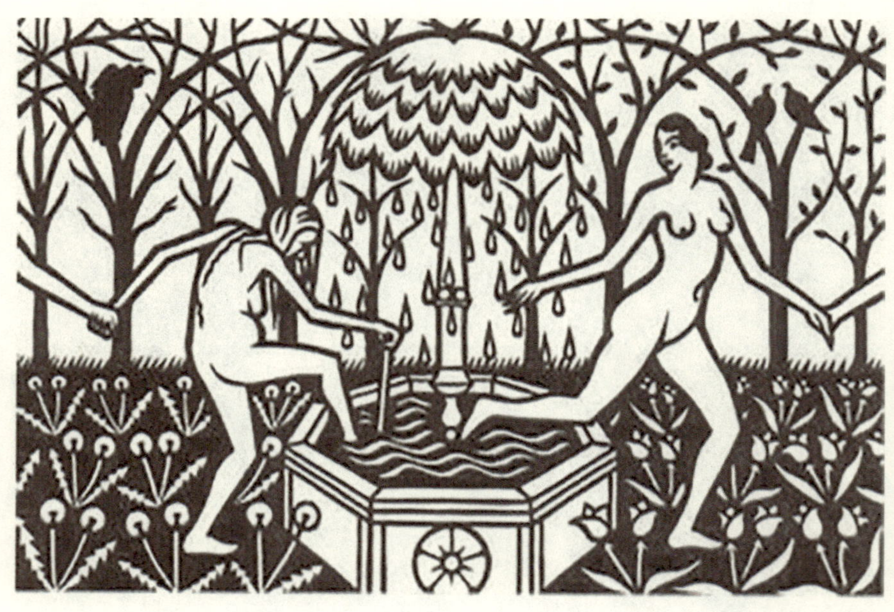

A rendering of a fountain of youth by the artist Joe Boruchow.

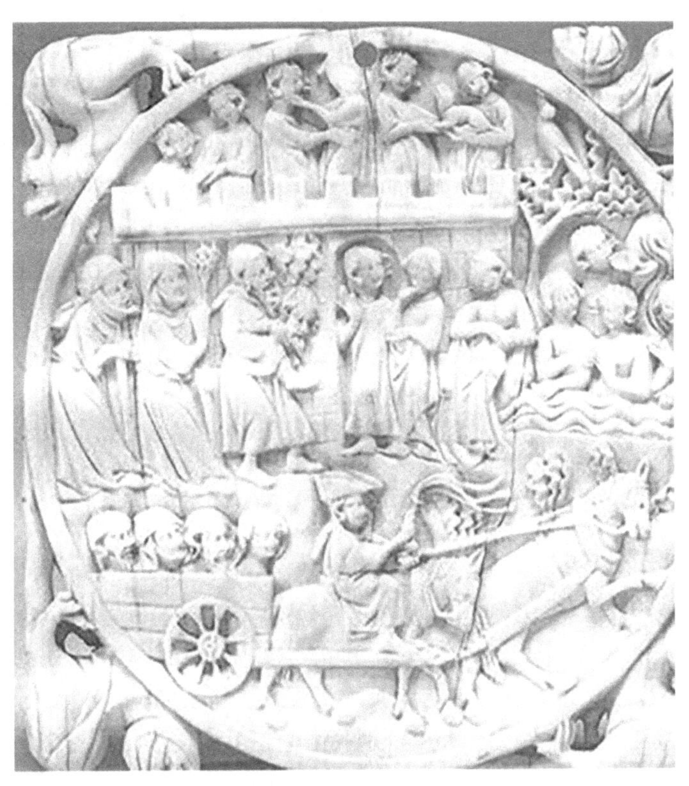

AD fourth century French ivory mirror case cover depicting a fountain of youth.

There are, however, no official original documents on Ponce de Leon expeditions to Florida, and the letters that he wrote to King Ferdinand never mentioned anything about fountains of youth. It appears that the stories and legends that inextricably link Ponce de Leon to fountains or rivers of youth are just stories and legends with no basis in fact.[6] Modern historians have debunked almost everything about those stories.

The uncertainties, the controversies, and the denials, however, did not stop the legends from enduring. There is a spring, for example, in St. Augustine, Florida, that to this day it is believed to be the actual fountain of youth discovered by Ponce de Leon in AD 1513. This fountain, which is located in the Archeological Park of St. Augustine (see photograph on the next page), is a very attractive and popular tourist destination, where older people come to regain their youth. Of course, no one does.

The irony with the fountain of St. Augustine is not only that its waters lack any magical powers, but also Ponce de Leon probably never set foot in St. Augustine.

Conclusion: Fountains of youth are just wishful thinking. What is a fact is that myriads of stories have been written claiming the existence of magical waters and linking the expeditions of Ponce de Leon to a quest for the fountain of youth. The actual discovery, however, of such a fountain by Ponce de Leon and its existence in St. Augustine is absolutely a myth with no basis in reality.

It appears that the only fountain of youth is in our brain. We, ourselves, are the source of the magical fountain.

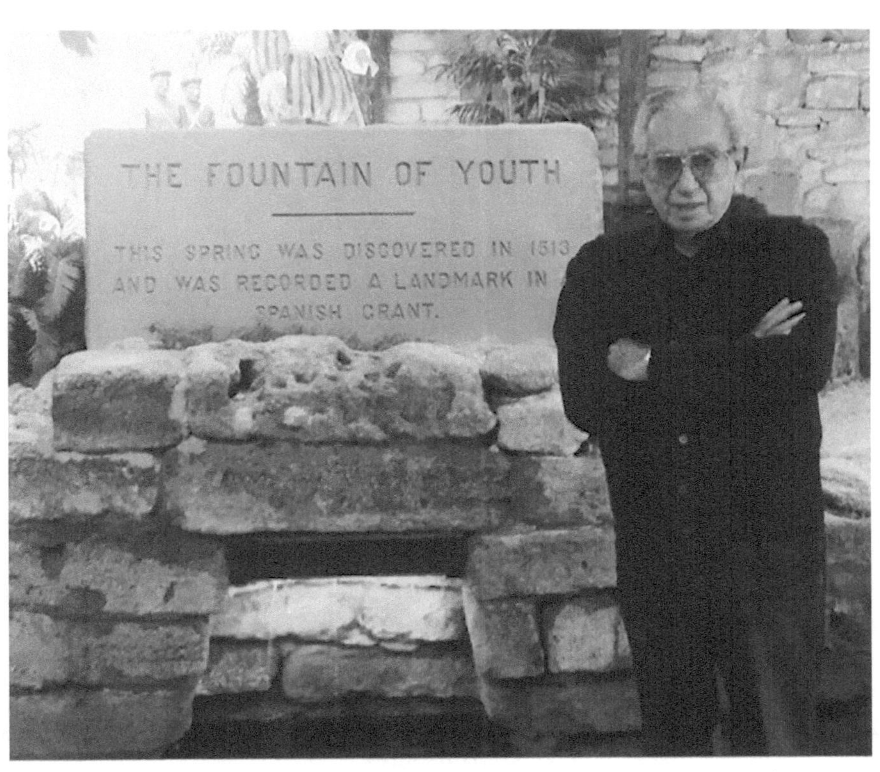

*The author in front of the alleged fountain of youth in the
Archeological Park of St. Augustine, Florida*

Elixir of Youth

Potions - Foods - Chemicals

The word "elixir" derives from the Arabic name "al iksir," which means miracle substance. According to its strict definition, "elixir of youth" is a mystical potion that grants the drinker eternal youth. The broader meaning of the term, however, covers diverse means that accomplish the same goal. They include potions, foods, drugs, exercises, genetic manipulations, and, perhaps inappropriately, cosmetics.

The quest for an elixir of youth consumed humanity for thousands of years across a wide spectrum of cultures. Several potions and foods were believed to possess the magic power to rollback the years and avert the frailty of aging.

In the Ancient Times

In Greece, mythology has it that the ancient Greek gods attained eternal youth and immortality by eating ambrosia and drinking nectar. Ambrosia, which was believed to derive from the horns of a magical goat, gave the gods power and strength and "made their body beautiful."

In China, many emperors attempted to achieve eternal youth by ingesting precious substances, such as "liquid gold"[7] or salts of mercury and arsenic, most of which were highly toxic and even lethal. There is a good possibility that several of those emperors died from elixir poisoning.

In India, the Hindu scriptures describe *amrit* as the nectar of immortality or *amrit ras* (immortality juice).

In Persia, their elixir was the *aab-i-hayat* (water of life).

All of these elixirs were products of the imagination of our ancient ancestors, and none of them had any basis in reality. Actually, perhaps we should not even call them elixirs since this term was not used until the seventh century AD.

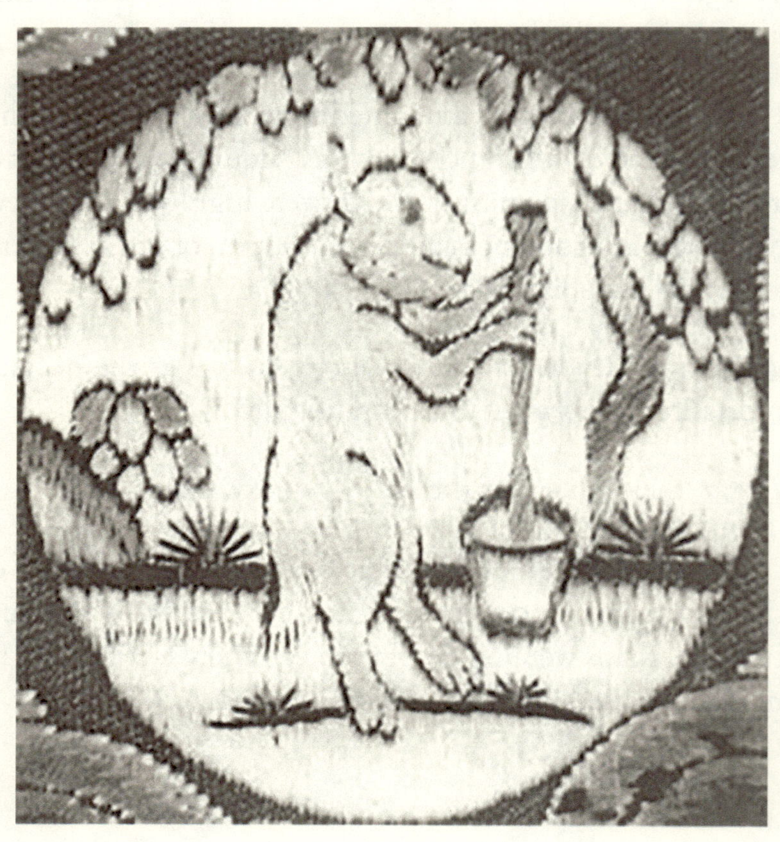

The mythological white hare preparing an elixir according to East Asian myth and folklore.

In Recent Times

New classes of agents have been claimed as potentially being capable of ameliorating aging. They include antioxidants, senolytic agents, hormones, and certain pharmaceuticals, such as rapamycine and metformin.

Antioxidants are agents that prevent the tissue-damaging effect of free radicals, an effect which is associated with aging (more details on free radicals and antioxidants are given in part 2 under "Good Nutrition"). Many articles and books have been written dealing with the effects of antioxidant dietary supplements. Some authors are skeptical and raise doubts on their efficacy and safety.[8] The predominant opinion, however, is that antioxidants are generally beneficial to health and contribute to the amelioration of aging.

Senolytic agents are chemicals that destroy senescent cells (aging cells) that accelerate the aging process. Senolytic compounds have been shown to slow the aging process in animals and to alleviate some symptoms of age-associated frailty in humans.

Metformin is a type II diabetes medicine that helps control blood sugar levels. It was reported that it also has anti-aging effects. In recent studies, it was shown to extend the life of mice. Clinical studies on human subjects are scheduled for the near future.

Rapamycine is an anticancer agent that is also claimed to possess anti-aging properties. It retarded multiple aspects of aging and increased the lifespan of animals.

Attempts to use *hormones* as elixirs of youth can be traced back to the nineteenth century AD, when Serge Voronoff, a French surgeon of Russian extraction, injected himself, in

1899, with extracts from dog and guinea pig testicles hoping to increase hormonal effects to retard aging.

There is no concrete evidence that any hormone can be considered as an elixir of youth. Some physicians, nevertheless, are prescribing human growth hormone (HGH) as an anti-aging agent. There are also many scam preparations and questionable products of replacement hormones that claim rejuvenating effects. Promotions of such products often use celebrity endorsements, which are very persuasive, particularly on the aging boomers.

In addition to estrogen and progesterone, other hormones, including testosterone, have been irresponsibly marketed by the anti-aging industry.

There are several agents that are currently being studied for potential anti-aging properties, including the senolytic preparations and metformin, which are very promising. If proven effective and safe in human studies, they will constitute a real and significant modern elixir of youth.

Exercises

Legend has it, that somewhere in the Himalayan Mountains of Tibet, monks passed down to several generations, spanning over 2,500 years, exercises with mystical powers that could preserve youth.

Allegedly, there is a group of lamas that discovered an elixir of youth and stories spread of old men who became healthy and full of vigor and virility after they entered a particular lamasery. The lamas described "five rites" (exercises) that improve health and invigorate.[9] Several people who practiced those rites claimed improved eyesight, memory, potency, hair growth, and generally anti-aging effects.[10] The benefits, however, that are most likely to be achieved by those exercises are increased energy and strength, clarity of thought, flexibility, and general improvement of well-being.[11]

Another form of rejuvenating exercises in the Far East is the *"DO-IN"* (dough-een), which consists of a series of self-massage techniques. These ancient exercises are also supposed to increase energy, clarity, and well-being.

In this category of rejuvenating exercises, we could also include yoga. This practice boasts to elevate consciousness, lower stress, and center the mind. Some people who practiced yoga for several decades often look much younger than their age.[12]

Genetic Manipulation

Scientists all over the world are studying the aging process in an attempt to find methods that would postpone the changes that trigger the ravages of aging. They found that the ends of chromosomes are capped by structures called telomeres that protect them from damage. As we age, the telomeres become progressively shorter, resulting in a diminution of their protective function. This, in turn, raises the odds of age-related failures, including development of Alzheimer's disease. Eventually, the erosion of the telomeres is so severe that the cell dies. The gradual erosion of the telomeres, however, is offset, to a certain degree, by an enzyme called telomerase which can rebuild the telomere caps. But as we age, this enzyme is inactivated.

In recent studies, scientists were able to administer a drug to prematurely aged mice and switch the telomerase back to life. The scientists expected that this technique would halt or slow the further aging of the animals. Instead, they were pleasantly surprised to observe that the treatment reversed the aging process. The animals were rejuvenated with the males regaining fertility[13] Genetic intervention is an exciting field of investigation with great potentials, but even though some progress has already been made, production of an agent for human use that would effectively prevent, delay, or reverse aging is probably many years away.

Conclusion: The myths and legends of the past are just that—myths and legends. The promises of the present may be fulfilled one day but, for the time being, are also just that—promises.

The products promoted by the anti-age industry as Elixirs of Youth, are of limited effectiveness, if any, and are mostly cosmetics claiming skin rejuvenation.

Advances in Gerontology, however, may eventually result in the discovery and production of real Elixirs of Youth. But that is for the future. In the meantime, my prescriptions for keeping young and for preventing memory failures, detailed in Part 2 and Part 3 of this book, may provide an immediate remedy for avoiding or, at least, delaying or ameliorating the frailty of old age.

PART 2

The Prescription for Longer Youth

Exercise

Think Young

Set Goals

The Prescription

Getting older should not automatically mean that we look and feel older or that we should slow down. There are ways to avert the frailties of aging and be active, vibrant, and look younger.

My prescription intends to provide instructions to hopefully attenuate the impact of accumulated years and provide a chance to live a little younger a little longer.

There are many factors that play a role in aging. Some of them, such as our genetic makeup, our DNA, or the effects of climate, are beyond our control. It is true that relatively recent gerontological studies provided a better understanding of the genetic control of aging and opened up new avenues of investigation with the potential of genetic engineering. Experiments on various living organisms have demonstrated that it is possible to induce gene mutations that influence aging and longevity.[14] Those studies, however, were conducted on low forms of life, and the results are preliminary. Sometime in the future, we may be able to manipulate our genes to delay aging, but at present, we are hostages of our genetic blueprint.

My prescription concerns factors that we can control. It deals with those significant factors that could influence the aging process but are subjugated to our will and to our determination. It involves precepts and guidelines that are relatively simple and easy to follow if there is motivation and willingness. Those precepts may require some changes in our habits and in our daily routine, but with determination and discipline, the changes can be adopted with no particular problems. It should be noted, however, that while most of the measures that are advocated are harmless, some of them may present risks for some people. Medical consultation is, therefore, advised before applying the recommended precepts and guidelines.

The prescription consists of three principal instructions:

1. MAINTAIN GOOD HEALTH

Good nutrition
No smoking
Alcohol in moderation
Regular medical checkups, preventive screening, and vaccinations
Adequate sleep
Exercise regularly

2. THINK YOUNG

3. DREAM AND SET GOALS

Let us discuss each of these instructions individually and see how they may affect the aging process.

Instruction No. 1

MAINTAIN GOOD HEALTH

Good Nutrition

Diets can have a considerable impact on the aging process. The amount and composition of food may affect complex interactions and produce appreciable changes in the functional consequences of aging. Balanced diets, with less calories and the right nutrients, can lessen the undesirable impact of aging on appearance and on function. Extreme diets, on the other hand, could affect aging adversely. Crash diets, for example, may produce irritability or depression and make us feel older by reducing our energy.

During normal aging, degenerative changes in the brain result in behavioral deficits manifested as impaired cognitive[15] and motor[16] functions. Impaired cognitive functions include memory deficits and other neurological disorders, such as Alzheimer's disease. Motor changes are manifested as impaired coordination and balance and decrease in muscular strength.

According to the "free radical* theory" of aging,[17] behavioral deficits are caused by oxidative action associated with free radicals that progressively damages tissues and organs and promotes aging. Antioxidants, by neutralizing the oxidative action of free radicals, exert a beneficial effect on aging. Fruits and vegetables that contain flavonoids ameliorate aging apparently because of their antioxidant properties.[18] Several epidemiologic studies suggest that diets with large amounts of fruits and vegetables may reduce the risk of Alzheimer's disease, and fruit and vegetable extracts have been shown to improve motor and cognitive behavior.[19,20] Also, cocoa, which contains flavonoids, was reported to slow age-related cognitive decline.[78] Apparently, plants synthesize chemical compounds with antioxidant and anti-inflammatory properties.[21,22]

There has been extensive research on the influence of various diets and nutrients on aging, including studies specifically on the effects of carbohydrates, proteins, lipids, vitamins, and minerals. The following is a short summary of the results and conclusions of these studies.

Carbohydrates The role of carbohydrates on aging is unclear, even though clinical studies have indicated that low-carbohydrate diets are generally beneficial for human health.[23] In general, low-caloric intake, referring primarily to low consumption of carbohydrates and fats, has a beneficial effect on aging. There

---

*　Free radicals are highly reactive atoms or groups of atoms that are products of normal metabolism.

have been reports that low-carbohydrate diets may delay aging[24] by preventing metabolic diseases and improving general health. It has also been shown that such diets lower levels of serum insulin, glucose, and triglycerides, which are implicated in aging and metabolic defects.[23]

Proteins There is no direct evidence linking protein intake to aging. It seems, however, that diets with animal protein may have a negative effect. In contrast, foods with plant protein may potentially be beneficial.

Lipids Regarding dietary lipids, it is well established that saturated fats and trans fats are generally detrimental to health[25]

On the other hand, polyunsaturated fats prevent aging-associated diseases and promote longevity.[25] Omega-3 fatty acids in fatty fish, such as salmon, lake trout, or tuna, and in nuts, such as walnuts, have been shown to have anti-aging effects.

Vitamins and minerals These are generally considered beneficial to health but seem to have little effect on aging.[26] Several studies conducted on a variety of animal species yielded controversial and contradictory results, possibly because of differences in the doses used.[27]

On the positive side, vitamins A, C, and E have been considered as having anti-aging effects because of their antioxidant properties.

It is nevertheless advisable to apply with caution the conventional view that vitamins delay aging.[25]

In view of the uncertainties and controversies regarding the influence of various nutrients on aging, it would be safe to conclude that dietary balance among various nutrients will have a greater impact on the process of aging than the effect of individual components.[28,29,30]

The following instructions regarding nutrition may be useful in reducing the effects of aging.

NUTRITIONAL ANTI-AGING INSTRUCTIONS

- Use healthy diets (Mediterranean diet)
- Use balanced diets
- Avoid crash diets
- Eat lots of fruits and vegetables
- Use polyunsaturated fats (olive oil)
- Eat foods with Omega-3 fats (salmon, tuna, lake trout, walnuts)
- Avoid saturated and trans fats (butter, fat, cream)
- Eat plant protein (legumes) rather than animal protein
- Reduce intake of calories (less fats and carbohydrates and, particularly, less sugar)
- Reduce intake of salt
- Drink plenty of water

It should be noted that for certain individuals, some of these instructions may be inappropriate, or even harmful, because of incompatibility with underlying medical conditions.

Consultation and advice from a physician should be sought before implementing them.

Conclusion: We should limit intake of calories; eat more fish, less meat, less butter, more olive oil, and plenty of fruits and veggies.

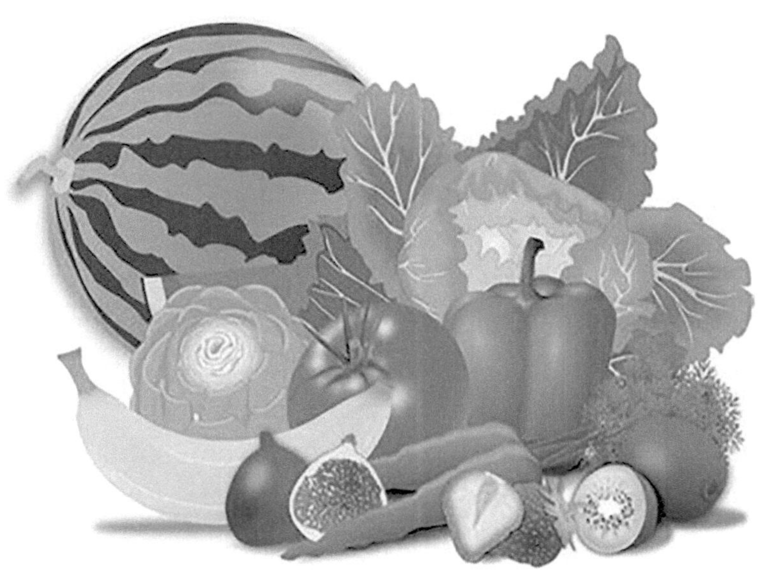

Eat Healthy Food

No Smoking

Smokers age at a faster rate than people who do not smoke. Smoking, in addition to its association with several detrimental health effects, including its implication in the pathogenesis of various cancers and cardiovascular diseases, also causes premature aging of the skin. Noticeable changes on the face and body appear as soon as 10 years after lighting up regularly.

Tobacco alters the appearance of skin, hair, and teeth in ways that add years to the looks of smokers who are often perceived much older than they actually are. This prematurely aged appearance of the skin is primarily due to the fact wrinkles that appear at an earlier age in people who smoke.

It had been reported that smokers in their 40s often have as many facial wrinkles as non-smokers in their 60s.

The more a person smokes, the greater the risk of premature wrinkling.[32]

Cigarette smoking causes aging of skin even more than exposure to sunlight. In fact, according to some studies, smoking and sunbathing at the same time is more dangerous than the combined effect of either culprit alone, and the risk for women is greater than for men.

Researchers have also found a link between smoking and accelerated loss of hair and graying.[33] It appears that cigarette smoking reduces the amount of nutrients that reach the hair leaving it lackluster and even discoloring it.

Smoking can impact aging in various ways including memory loss, aging of the skin, bad breath, and "smoker's tobacco scent."

The following are changes that contribute to the aged appearance of smokers:

Wrinkles
Sagging of the skin
Gray complexion
Loss of natural glow
Gaunt look
Yellow teeth
Dull and less vibrant skin, hair, nails

There are still questions as to how precisely smoking exerts its damaging effect on the skin. Results from several studies indicate that the nicotine in the cigarettes causes vasoconstriction, which narrows the lumen of capillaries and arterioles in the superficial layers of the skin. This, in turn, results in a decreased blood flow and reduced supply of nutrients and oxygen to the tissues of the skin. Contributing to the reduction of oxygen may also be the possible displacement of tissue oxygen by carbon monoxide contained in cigarette smoke.

In addition to depriving the skin of oxygen and nutrients, tobacco smoke damages the tissues through chemical interactions. It contains more than four thousand chemicals, many of which, including nicotine, cause degradation of collagen and elastin, which are the connective tissue fibers of the skin that give it strength and elasticity. As a result, the skin sags and wrinkles.

According to some in vitro studies, smoking causes this degradation of the connective tissue of the skin by increasing the production of an enzyme that breaks down collagen and elastic fibers.[34,35]

With all the unappealing manifestation of premature tobacco-induced aging, one wonders how is it possible for anyone to continue smoking in a society that values youth. This is particularly amazing regarding women, who are so concerned and self-conscious of their appearance. It will not be surprising if, for some smokers, awareness of the undesirable changes in their physical appearance is a stronger incentive to quit smoking than the risk of cancer or cardiovascular diseases. An international study found that 13.3 percent of men and 21 percent of women acknowledge that the effect of smoking on their appearance was one of the factors that motivated them to quit.[36] In a UK study, young adults aged sixteen through twenty-four also took their appearance into consideration in making the decision to quit smoking.[37] Also in a UK study, women aged eighteen through twenty-four were shocked when they were shown (using special software) their future appearance if they continue to smoke. Those pictures with the unappealing old-looking faces significantly increased their motivation to stop smoking.[38,39]

Conclusion: Smoking promotes aging with the most striking impact on the skin. We should not smoke and should quit if we do.

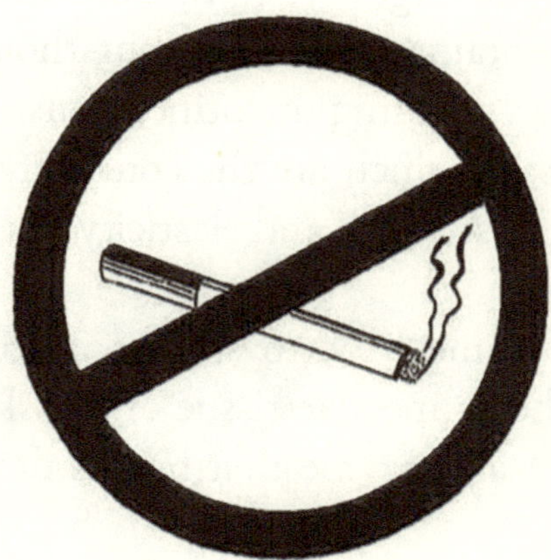

Do Not Smoke

Alcohol in Moderation

The effect of alcohol on aging depends on the amount and frequency of drinking. It should be noted that older individuals are more sensitive to alcohol. The same amount that can be harmless, or even beneficial, to a young person may have ill effects on an older individual. Excessive use of alcohol can promote aging. The National Institute of Alcohol Abuse and Alcoholism found that alcoholism may accelerate normal aging or cause premature aging of the brain.[40] Symptoms of aging may also appear at the appropriate time but in a more exaggerated form.[41]

In people with dermatological issues, alcohol may have more harmful effects, causing a flare and worsening of the skin condition.

Consumption of moderate amounts of alcohol, on the other hand, may be beneficial.

According to the U.S. Government Dietary Guidelines, "moderate level" of drinking means up to one drink per day for women and up to two drinks per day for men. The definition of "drink" is as follows:

For wine, one drink equals five fluid ounces.
For beer, one drink equals twelve fluid ounces.
For hard liquor,[*] one drink equals one and half fluid ounces.

Particularly beneficial for attenuating the manifestations of aging is the red wine, consumed, however, in moderate amounts and by healthy individuals. This preference to red wine may be

---

* Hard liquor refers to 80-proof distilled liquor.

because it contains antioxidants that counteract some of the oxidative processes involved in aging.

Conclusion: Drinking should be in moderation and preferably red wine.

Regular Medical Checkups and Preventive Screening

Regular Medical Checkups

The reason for including regular medical checkups and preventive screening in my prescription is that good health is a prerequisite for staying young and active. In most cases, it would be unreasonable to expect people to act and look young, to be vibrant and energetic, if they are sick or suffering from chronic debilitating conditions.

The rationale of this justification is based on the assumption that regular medical checkups and preventive screening contribute to the maintenance of good health.

The validity of this assumption, however, has been challenged. Results from relatively recent studies indicate that general medical checkups are not effective in preserving health and, consequently, do not support their use by the general population.[42]

An international group that reviews scientific evidence conducted recently a meta-analysis of randomized trials involving 182,880 patients, one group of which had medical checkups and another group did not.[43] The medical checkups did not influence the patient's health or longevity. Patients in the checkup group died from heart disease and cancer at the same rate as their peers who did not have checkups.

Of course, such analysis yields only averaged data for a large group of people, not for an individual person. It is possible that some types of patients could be benefited from medical checkups and other types may not. Patients who are healthy and in good shape may not need regular annual checkups. The American Medical Association and other similar organizations also moved away from the yearly checkup.[47] They recommend "periodic health assessments" to be performed every five years for young individuals and at shorter intervals for older people.

Furthermore, some critics point out that yearly medical checkups of healthy individuals could lead to unnecessary tests, some of which could cause complications. Also, some tests may even be harmful because they often yield false positive results, requiring further tests, and also because they cause patients needless anguish.

Some other physicians and medical organizations, on the other hand, maintain that regular medical checkups and tests are needed because they can detect warning signs of health problems, such as high blood pressure, high blood sugar, or increased cholesterol, and provide an opportunity to take measures to prevent them from developing into chronic diseases. Or they can help catch early serious health problems, like initial stages of cancers, aneurisms[*], and heart disease, when chances for cure are better.

Periodic medical examinations have been advocated since the 1920s.[44] Many studies have been done since, many opinions have been expressed, but the issue is still unsettled. Doctors continue to debate the value of regular annual medical checkups.[47, 77] Some want them abandoned, others feel they are important and should be practiced.

It is interesting that many private insurance companies, and even Medicare, include annual medical checkups in their coverage.

So how then does one proceed in the middle of this uncertainty and unending controversy?

As I said earlier, regular annual medical checkups for some individuals may be of value, for some others may not. "One size fits all" should certainly not apply here. Young healthy

----

[*]   Aneurism is a bulge in an artery that weakens its wall.

individuals probably do not need regular annual checkups. Periodic regular examinations for older people and for certain more vulnerable groups, however, might be a wiser approach. But when should these periodic regular medical checkups start, and how often should they be performed?

There is even less consensus regarding the required frequency of these regular checkups. The issue is complicated by the fact that parallel to the regular checkups, it is recommended that patients undergo preventive screenings, which are initiated at different ages and repeated at different intervals. There is also the question of what do we mean by "regular" checkups. The moment a medical problem pops up, the checkup ceases to be regular.

Despite all these complexities and controversies, attempts were made to come up with some compromising but realistic suggestions.

The American Medical Association's recommendation to perform periodic health assessments every five years for ages eighteen through forty, and one to three years for people over forty, seems a reasonable approach. The suggestion to determine the appropriate frequency of medical checkups on the basis of age, sex, medical condition, and risk factors for each patient[45] might even be better. Also, the parameters that impact on the desired frequency of medical checkups perhaps should also include family history and lifestyle.

Preventive Screening

In addition to the regular medical checkups, protection of health requires preventive screening for the early detection of serious and potentially life-threatening medical problems, such as malignancies, cardiovascular disorders, aneurisms, and diabetes.

Early detection by screening procedures is important because, as it was mentioned earlier regarding regular medical checkups, it provides an opportunity for easier and more effective treatment.

The screening tests are initiated at different ages and repeated periodically at intervals depending on the nature of the test, the risk factors, and the condition of the patient.

The screening procedures that are recommended by various health organizations include:

Colonoscopy: For lesions of the colon (large intestine), including cancer, polyps, and diverticulosis (a pouch in the wall of the intestine). Early detection of polyps is important because some of them, if left alone, progress into full-blown cancer.

Fecal occult blood test: For bleeding in the gastrointestinal tract. A positive test may indicate the presence of malignancy, ulcers, and other lesions in the stomach or in the intestines.

Mammography: For breast cancer.

Pap smear: For cervical cancer, which is easy to treat when caught early.

Bone density test: For osteoporosis (porous bones). This test is particularly recommended for women who, after menopause, are more vulnerable to loss of minerals from their bones, making them weaker and more friable.

Blood pressure measurements: For hypertension (high blood pressure), which is called the "silent killer" because one can have it and not be aware of it. Hypertension can cause heart attacks, stroke, and kidney and eye problems.

Cholesterol determination: For cardiovascular disease. This test usually measures total cholesterol and high- and low-density lipoproteins, known as good and bad cholesterol. High levels, particularly of bad cholesterol, may lead to heart attack or stroke.

Abdominal ultrasound: For the detection of abdominal aortic aneurism (AAA), which is a bulge in the wall of the main abdominal artery. Also silent, this lesion, is more common in men who smoked at any point in their lives. Aneurisms progressively increase in size and become life-threatening because, if not treated early, they can rupture and cause fatal bleeding.

Serum glucose determination: For type II diabetes (high blood sugar). If not controlled, diabetes can cause complications, including blindness, kidney disease, and damage in the limbs that may require amputation.

Skin inspection: For growths, some of which can be serious, like melanoma, which is a malignant, life-threatening lesion.

Vaccinations

The framework of preventive health care should also include immunizations, which are vital for preventing or lessening the severity of diseases.

Seasonal flu vaccine: Protection from influenza.

Pneumonia vaccine: Protection from lung infection.

<u>*Shingles vaccine:*</u> Protection from a viral skin disease manifested with pain and a rash of small blisters.

<u>*Tetanus immunization:*</u> Protection from infectious disease contracted through a cut or wound, causing muscular contractions and spasm of jaw (lockjaw).

The tables that follow show the age of initiation and the frequency of screening procedures and vaccinations recommended, for most part, by the U.S. Preventing Services Task Force (USPSTF).[*]

---

[*]   The American Cancer Society recommends cancer-related checkups every three years for twenty through forty-year-olds and annually for those older than forty.

PREVENTIVE SCREENING

PROCEDURE	INITIATION AT	REPEAT
Colonoscopy	50	50-75 every 10 years
Fecal occult blood	50	Annually
Mammography	50	50-74 every 2 years
Pap smear	18	18-39 every 3 years
Bone density	60	40-64 every 5 years
Blood Pressure (BP)	18	With normal BP, every 2 years With high BP, annually
Cholesterol Test	20	20-35 every 4-6 years Over 35 depends
Abdominal ultrasound	65	One-time screening
Serum glucose (if high BP)		Depends
Skin inspection	19	19-49 every 3 years Over 49 annually

VACCINATIONS

VACCINATIONS	INITIATION AT	REPEAT
Flu vaccine	6m	Annually
Pneumonia vaccine	65	One time
Shingles vaccine	60	One time
Tetanus immunization	7	Booster every 10 years

Conclusion: We should have the medical exams, tests, and vaccinations that our physicians recommend.

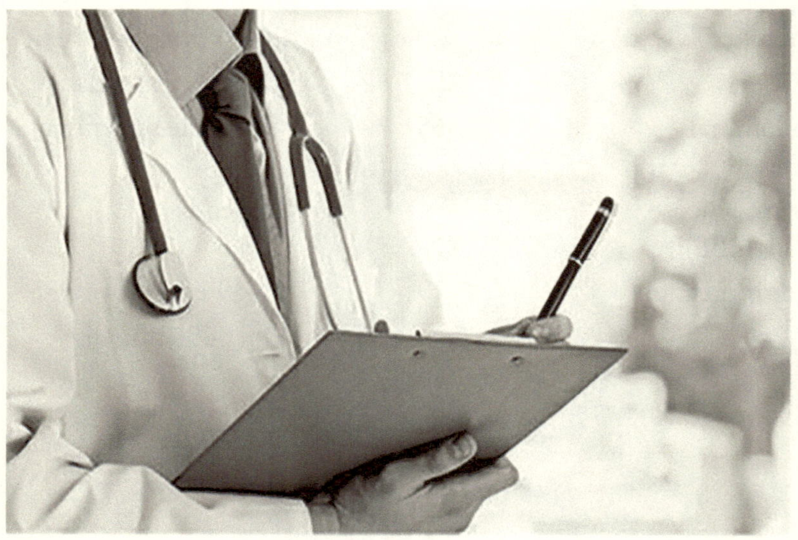

Have Medical Checkups

Adequate Sleep

Night Sleep

A good night's sleep is important for keeping young. It is essential in maintaining good health, which, in turn, is a prerequisite for reducing the effects of aging. Sleep deprivation may disrupt hormonal balance, hinder metabolism, and accelerate the onset and severity of aging, including loss of memory and problems with thinking and focusing.

In developed countries, the average amount of sleep has been declining since the beginning of the last century. Busy jobs, sports, entertainment, and other activities of the modern world consume most of our day at the expense of sleeping time. The average duration of sleep from nine hours per night at the beginning of the twentieth century fell to eight to eight and a half hours in the 1960s and 1970s and to seven to seven and a half hours in the past few years.

According to most medical authorities, young adults should sleep seven to nine hours and older people seven to eight hours per night. The notion that old people do not need much sleep may not be correct.

In view of the necessity for adequate healthy sleep, attention has been drawn to the fact that many people have trouble sleeping. According to the National Sleep Foundation, nearly 62 percent of American adults experience a sleep problem a few nights each week. There is a great variety of reasons for this problem. Behavior and lifestyle can have a major impact on the induction, duration, and quality of sleep. Our habits and daily routines, the food we eat, the drinks we consume, the medications we take, how we spend our evenings, pressures at work, family issues, and illnesses can all make a good night's sleep elusive. We may not be able to control all those interfering factors, but if we could make some adjustments and adopt certain healthy sleep habits, we could be able to avoid problems with insomnia.

The following is a list of sleep habits that can help us achieve adequate healthy sleep.

HEALTHY SLEEP HABITS

Maintain a consistent sleep-wake schedule. Go to bed and wake up the same time every day, even in weekends, holidays, and vacation. Keeping the same sleeping routine regulates the body's clock and helps us fall asleep and stay asleep.

Keep the bedroom comfortable. Cool, quiet, and dark.

Use comfortable mattress and pillows.

Use the bedroom for sleeping only. Do not eat or watch TV in the bedroom. Do not use electronics (laptops, cell phones) in bed. Such activities may excite us or cause stress or anxiety that may make it difficult to fall and remain asleep.

Practice regular relaxing bedtime rituals. Take a warm bath or shower, read a book, listen to soothing music. Relaxing pre-sleep routines tell our body it is time to go to sleep.

Go to bed only when we are truly tired and sleepy. If we are not sleeping after twenty minutes, we should get out of bed, go to another room, and do something relaxing.

Do not have large meals before bedtime. Do not go to bed stuffed, but do not go to sleep hungry. Have small snacks.

Avoid caffeine and nicotine in late afternoon and evening. They are stimulants that may interfere with sleep.

Avoid alcohol. It may induce sleep but interrupts it later.

Visit the bathroom. We should empty our bladder before we go to sleep.

Exercise regularly. But not too close to bedtime.

Napping

To nap or not to nap? This is the question! Yes, this has been the question for quite some time. Should we take naps? And would an afternoon siesta help ameliorate undesirable aging manifestation?

This issue of nap desirability has long been debated and is still controversial. Before I discuss the pros and cons, however, let me take a position up front and respond to the question "to nap or not to nap" with a resounding yes, "to nap." Yes, we should take siestas.

Those who are against napping argue that it has several drawbacks, such as grogginess and disorientation after waking up from a nap and interference with the normal nighttime sleep. They speculate that napping may disrupt the normal circadian[*] rhythm of the body, resulting in a reduction in the duration or in the quality of nocturnal sleep.

Some studies have gone as far as to suggest that napping is linked to ill health. This association could be interpreted, however, as the napping being the result and not the cause of illness. Because of such unfavorable reports, several scientists and health organization advised against taking naps. The American Academy of Sleep Medicine, for example, placed on its website the message "Avoid taking naps if you can."

---

*   Circadian refers to a twenty-four-hour cycle of physiologic processes.

On the other side of the fence, numerous studies contradict the negative reports and conclude that napping exerts many beneficial effects, including

Improved alertness
Better memory
Reduced fatigue
Relaxation
Better mood
Improved mental function
Enhanced cognitive performance
Supplementation of insufficient night sleep

There is evidence from a variety of sources that daytime snoozing does not interfere with nocturnal sleep. In one study on healthy men and women aged fifty-five through eighty-eight years (average seventy years), it was shown that napping had no impact on subsequent nighttime sleep quality or duration, resulting in a significant increase in the total twenty-four-hour sleep amounts.[48] This is important, considering the fact that older individuals may not be capable of sleeping more than six hours per twenty-four-hour period.

The lack of interference of daytime napping with nocturnal sleep also receives support by some ancillary data, such as observations that napping is more common in older adults who sleep well at night than in those who don't.

In attempting to reconcile the pros and cons of napping, let me point out that the contradictory results may be because of differences in the age of the studied populations and in the duration of napping. Long siestas may have drawbacks, but short naps could be beneficial. Also, napping may have ill effects on younger adults but a positive influence on older individuals. A study on the population of the Greek island Ikaria (the Greek study) showed that the benefits of napping increased with age. Negative effects were seen in participants forty to fifty years old, but in older subjects (average seventy years), napping had no detrimental effect on nighttime sleep duration or quality.[49]

It is recommended that naps be short, no more than thirty minutes for young adults and no more than sixty minutes for the elderly. It should be pointed out, however, that napping, even for just a few minutes, is beneficial. Naps should be taken in the afternoon (2:00–3:00 p.m.) when we experience post-lunch sleepiness, and the siesta is less likely to interfere with nighttime sleep. Like with nocturnal sleep, the room should be quiet, dark, with a comfortable temperature and no distractions.

Conclusion: The preponderance of evidence indicates that we can enjoy the anti-aging effects of napping, including enhanced memory and alertness, better mood, and quicker reactions, without affecting the onset, duration, or quality of nighttime sleep. We should nap.

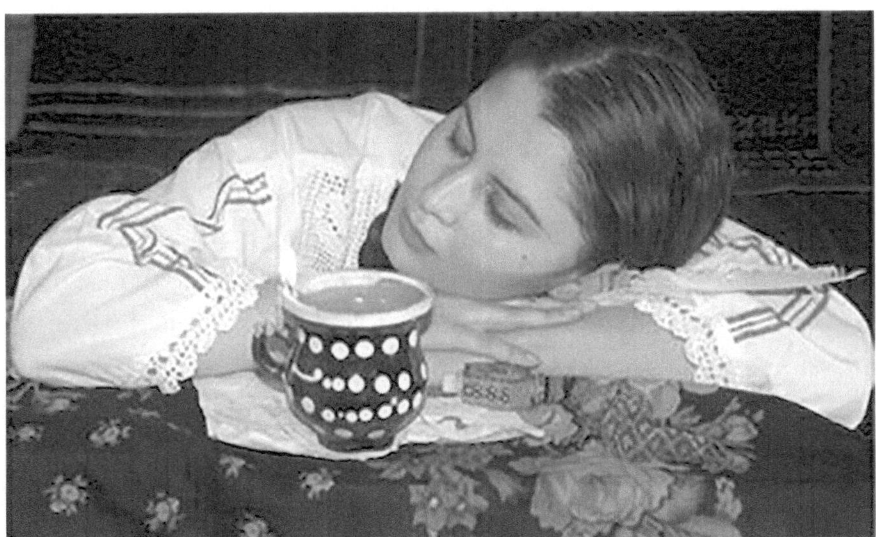

Take A Nap

Exercise Regularly

Regular exercise is the most important component of my prescription. It is essential for staying young. It is a sine qua non. Why is exercise so important?

As we are getting older, certain processes in our brain progressively deteriorate, resulting in a decline of physiological functions, including impaired motor performance and cognitive deficits.[50,51] Reductions in functional capacity of the aged can generally be attributed to loss of cardiovascular, respiratory, neuromuscular, and metabolic functions that typically occur with aging.[52] The manifestations of these functional declines may include memory loss, Alzheimer's disease, reduced muscular strength, and impaired coordination and balance. This age-related deterioration in the capacities of the various physiological systems results in a decreased ability of older individuals to perform common activities of daily living.[52]

Because of the dramatic increase of the aging population, particularly in the Western societies, great interest was generated in investigating the possibility that changes in the lifestyle of aging people could prevent, ameliorate, or even reverse their functional decline. Numerous multidisciplinary studies that have been conducted both on human subjects and on animals have convincingly demonstrated that physical exercise can indeed ameliorate and even reverse the age-related decline of physiological functions.

In studies with adult animals, small amounts of exercise was sufficient to completely reverse infection-induced impairment of long-term memory,[53] and treadmill exercise improved short-term memory in aged animals.[54]

Other experiments on aging animals showed that moderate exercise produced improved performance in behavioral tests of neuromuscular function.[51]

It is interesting that these experiments also revealed that the activities of antioxidant enzymes in the brain of aged animals decrease and that exercise prevents this reduction in the antioxidant activity.

It was concluded from those studies that moderate exercise triggers regulatory responses that retard some age-dependent processes, such as the impairment of behavioral performances.[51]

Studies on human subjects also produced encouraging results regarding alleviation of both motor and cognitive deficits of aging.

It was shown in controlled studies that six months of moderate aerobic exercise (moderate walking) could reliably reverse age-related cognitive decline.[50] This beneficial effect of aerobic exercise on cognitive function was greater for tasks of executive control, such as task coordination, planning, working memory, maintenance of goals, and task switching. Meta-analysis on many intervention studies provided corroborative evidence that fitness training improves executive control processes.[55] Regular exercise and an active lifestyle during adulthood have been associated with reduced risk and protective effects for mild cognitive impairment and Alzheimer's disease.[56]

There have also been reports that physical activity produces a feeling of psychological well-being. It was proposed that this effect is mediated through the observed significant increases in endogenous opioids following exercise.[57] Regarding the effects of exercise on age-associated decline in motor performance, it has been reported that exercise can reverse or at least slow this decline.[58]

The beneficial effects of exercise on the mobility and independence of older people are very important because to feel and to act young, we need freedom of movement and functional independence. Impaired balance and gait are the two most significant risk factors for limited mobility and for falls in the elderly.[59,60,61,62]

The beneficial effect of physical exercise on age-related functional deficits was attributed to improvements in the efficiency of the capillary system and increases in oxygen supply to the brain, resulting in an enhancement of metabolic activity and oxygen intake in nerve tissue.[56] Increase in cerebral metabolic activity was also considered as the possible mechanism in the observed significant improvement in neuropsychological test scores by aerobic exercises.[63]

Exercise also helps get rid of "emotional toxins" from anger, frustration, anxieties, sorrow, and stress, all of which promote aging. There are reports that major depression, whether in the past or present, may actually speed up the aging process at the molecular level.[64] Findings presented in the journal *Thorax*, a specialist publication of the *British Medical Journal*, showed that people who constantly feel anger are more likely to age quicker,[65] and chronic stress was consider a factor in premature aging, producing worried face, facial wrinkles, and slower movement.[69] Exercise was reported to counteract the aging-promoting effects of depression,[66,67] anxiety[67-68], and stress.[67]

Now that we have reviewed the importance of physical exercise in preventing, reversing, or attenuating the undesirable effects of aging, let us see how much exercise we need. According to federal guidelines, adults need thirty minutes of exercise per day for five days to a total of one hundred fifty minutes per week. It is understood that for elderly people, this goal may be too hard to reach.

The good news is that recent studies have shown that even fifteen minutes a day, five days a week, make an appreciable difference.

Many people avoid physical exercise, not so much because of aging or health limitations and restrictions, but rather because of inertia, inconvenience, and resistance to lifestyle changes. Such people bring all sorts of excuses for not engaging in physical exercises: busy schedules, lack of time, getting old, inability to afford a membership to a gym, or the purchase of exercising equipment. You do not necessarily need a gym. You can walk! Walking is a good exercise. You can park one block or two short of your destination and walk. Or you can climb one or two flights of stairs.

People don't fail to exercise because they are getting older.
They are getting older because they fail to exercise.

Conclusion: As I said in the beginning of this section, exercise is the most pivotal component of my prescription. It is a lifestyle factor that can lead to enhanced physical and mental health throughout life and keep us a little younger a little longer. We should exercise regularly and consistently.

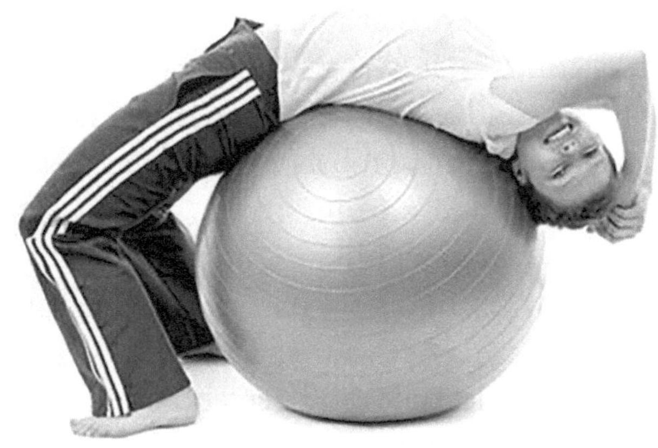

EXERCISE, EXERCISE!

Instruction No. 2

THINK YOUNG

Aging is a self-fulfilling expectation. Most of us inherited the old notion that as we age, our minds and our bodies deteriorate. We have been led to believe that aging is associated with physical and mental decline, that we will experience progressively diminished motor and cognitive functions. Those who are entering their senior years probably heard the well-meaning but pessimistic advice and warnings:

"From now on, it is downhill."

"You should not get into new ventures at your age." "Now you should take it easy." "Act your age."

As a result of these attitudes and perceptions of aging, senior years are viewed as time to take it easy and slow down. It was reported, for example, that as people age, they consider exercise increasingly inappropriate.[40] This thinking is unfortunate because how we perceive aging can influence how we age. Recent studies have shown that the way we think impacts the way we feel and determines our behavioral pattern. Thoughts, expectations, and perceptions are linked to neurological, biochemical, and physiological processes that generate our actions and behavior. If we perceive aging as time for an inevitable reduction in activities, in other words, if we "think old," our lifestyle will be downgraded, encouraging a physical decline. On the other hand, if we think younger than we are, if we adopt a younger self-image, we will start to feel young, and we will behave young.

The hypothetical situation I am describing below is far-fetched and completely unrealistic, but I am using it to stress the impact the perception of our age has on our lives.

Let us say you are seventy-nine years old and you are presented with convincing evidence that a mistake was made and the date of birth on your birth certificate is wrong. According to the corrected documents, you are not seventy-nine—you are only fifty-nine years old. Do you think this revision of your age would make any difference in your life? Would your actions and behavior change now that you learned that you are only fifty-nine years old? Would you be more youthful? I bet you would. Most people would. You would definitely be transformed to a more youthful and vibrant individual because the restrictive influence of the seventy-nine calendar years would no longer be there.

The potential to live like a younger individual existed, but it was suppressed by the weight of those seventy-nine calendar years. Our biological age may be that of a younger person, we may feel younger (most people do), but unfortunately, we have been conditioned to think and live not as we feel but as our calendar age dictates.

The message that I intended to convey with this hypothetical story is that to enjoy a youthful life, we have to think young.

Our brain, with its ability to form new synapses*,has to reassess the situation, change outlook, and reprogram the commands it sends to our body in order to alter behavioral patterns.

It is possible, of course, that because of the wear and tear of so many years, the body may send to the brain messages of inability to comply with the new commands and, thus, hinder their implementation. But let us not underestimate the power of the brain over the rest of the body. In studies of the brain-body interactions, it has been shown that mental processes can affect the body's physiology and alter outcomes.[71] When we see that the desired outcomes are attainable, we continue to aim for those outcomes.[72] Once we realize that we are able to enjoy a more youthful life, we will strive to preserve it.

When we think young, the brain, through neurotransmitters, sends out impulses that by energizing muscles, by activating the endocrine system and the release of hormones, and by mobilizing the participation of the autonomic nervous system, stimulates functions that give us vitality. We feel, we act, and we look young. And the younger we look, the younger we feel, and feeling younger reflects again on our expression. Our eyes glitter, our face glows, we exhibit a youthful luster. Our talk and walk are becoming free and vibrant. We feel sure of ourselves, and we behave with an effervescent disposition. Our lifestyle changes. We socialize more and become more involved and more active. We get up in the morning eager and energetic. We set tasks and goals for ourselves, and we look at the future with confidence and anticipation.

To contrast the mentality of those who *think young* from those who do not, and to give the issue a realistic down-to-earth

---

* Synapse is a neural connection; a junction between nerve cells in order to transmit signals.

dimension, let me cite to you a personal experience I had with people who *do not think young.*

> *Twenty five years ago, I attended, with my wife Gaby, a class reunion at the Pallini Beach Hotel, a very nice seaside summer resort in Greece.*
>
> *My wife and I were pleased this resort was selected for the reunion because we both love tennis and the resort has many tennis courts.*
>
> *In the late afternoon, while I was talking to a group of classmates, Gaby came to me and announced, "I made tennis reservations for eight o'clock."*
>
> *One of my classmates who heard the announcement asked, "Whom is Gaby going to play tennis with?"*
>
> *"With me," I replied.*
>
> *"With you?" wondered the classmate. "You play tennis? At your age?"*

And I was only sixty-five years old at that time. Poor classmate. He thought sixty-five was too old to play tennis. He was not "thinking young," and so were also the others in the group because their silence indicated that they agreed with him. Is it not a pity that their notions and misconceptions of aging deprived them of living a fuller and more youthful life? They were not sick or disabled. Most of them were in the same physical shape that I was. They could play tennis if they wanted to.

I played tennis then, and I still play tennis now—twenty-five years later! Studies on subjects that were followed for an eighteen-year-period have shown that those with a more positive self-perception of aging had a better functional health than those with a more negative perception.[73]

The question now is, how do we change our self-perception of aging? How do we bring ourselves to "think young"?

Becoming conscious of the prevailing assumptions regarding aging is a good start. Let us then tell ourselves that those assumptions are false and misleading. Let us be aware that mental and physical decline are not inevitable as we grow older. We should let go of the current mind-set. We must abandon the misperceptions of aging and adopt a younger self-image and a positive attitude. Our state of mind, our desires, and our thoughts are very powerful tools for influencing the rate at which we age. Most people, I believe, are able to "think young" without special assistance. There are, however, mind-body techniques that may provide some help to achieve the desired mind settings. One such simple technique that may be helpful in acquiring a new state of mind is repeatedly writing down affirmations. In our case, for example, to write out the words "I am young" over and over for a week or two. The mere act of writing out such words again and again for several days may help us break through old thought patterns and negativity that are hampering us from realizing full psychobiological potentials.[74]

Conclusion: Aging does not automatically mean a physical and mental decline. By thinking young, we may be able to avoid or even reverse the effects of aging and live a more youthful and vibrant life.

Instruction No. 3

DREAM AND SET GOALS

As it was mentioned in previous sections, aging is associated with a progressive motor and cognitive decline. It was also mentioned that this functional deterioration that we experience as we are getting old could be delayed, reduced, or even reversed with exercise, proper diet, and maintenance of good health. The preceding section emphasized the pivotal role of "thinking young" in counteracting the effects of aging. Instructions 1 and 2 already dealt with those issues. This section will present another factor that I believe has a profound effect on aging: dreaming and setting goals.

If we want to stay young, we should continue to dream and set consecutive goals, goals that follow one after another, in our lives. We should set successive targets for our future. They can be short-term or long-term goals, big as well as trivial goals, performance goals or learning goals. Let me give some examples to illustrate what the terms "goals" and "targets" refer to in the context of this section.

Fixing our closet tomorrow, seeing our children or grandchildren, or entertaining our friends on the coming weekend are examples of short-term goals. They are rather trivial goals. Nevertheless, for the potential effect that they may have on aging, they are important. The goals can also be more ambitious, like planning a cruise to the Greek islands next summer, buying a new car, or expanding our business.

In the examples given above, the goals are performance goals. Equally important are learning goals, such as learning a new language or a new skill.

One of the most disturbing shortcoming in aging is the cognitive decline and, particularly, the loss of memory and the more serious and alarming Alzheimer's disease. According to the Alzheimer's Association, more than five million people over sixty-five are suffering from Alzheimer's disease in the United States. Experts predict that by the year 2025, this number may exceed seven million.

Recent studies demonstrated that goals and challenges improve cognitive health. Goals and goal-related processes have been shown to motivate behavior both in terms of isolated cognitive tasks and general life desires.[43] The motivation and the effort to reach a set target helps seniors maintain their mental health. Goal-setting even seems to boost self-efficacy and buffer the negative effects of lower confidence levels found in older adults.[43]

People without life goals, without aspirations, they are not only getting old, they are also practically dormant. They don't live; they only exist. Having dreams, setting goals, gives us purpose in life, *raison d'etre*.

Looking forward to reaching a target, the preparation, the anticipation, the following of the progress that has been attained are all exciting and stimulating. The effort to reach our targets keeps us occupied and alert. This, in turn, fights boredom that often plagues seniors and is known to promote aging. The mental and somatic activities involved in pursuing goals elicit a sense of well-being that gives us a vibrant disposition and makes us act, feel, and look young.

Conclusion: Dreaming, setting successive goals and targets will help us stay young.

PART 3

The Prescription for a
Better Memory

Memory and Forgetfulness

Introduction

The tremendous progress in medicine in recent decades, resulted in a significant increase of our life expectancy. This welcomed prolongation of life, however, also brought several age-related problems. One of them is lapses of memory which become more frequent and more pronounced as we enter our golden years.

Memory is a unique and vital faculty of the brain. It is an essential function for the normal performance of routine daily activities. It is a *sine qua non*. Serious memory loss could impact activities that we don't even suspect would be affected. It would be impossible, for example, to understand this book as you read it right now. Paragraphs will make no sense unless when you read their end you remember what they said at their beginning.

Memory is not perfect. Most of us, sooner or later, we will experience some memory problem. The problem may be insignificant, like that of Peter who, sometimes, forgets where he left his reading glasses or his car keys. Or, it could be serious, like that of Maria, who does not remember where the toilet is.

Even worse would be the case of Margaret who does not remember that to empty her bladder she has to go to the toilet!

One of the most common memory problems is our inability to remember recent information or experiences. We cannot remember, for instance, where we parked the car, or why did we walk into the kitchen. And, sometimes we wonder how come we can recall childhood experiences but we forget events that took place only a few days ago. We do not remember, hypothetically, the name of the professor from Harvard who was introduced to us only the day before yesterday, but we do remember the name of the teacher we had in elementary school man years go. This apparent paradox will be easy to explain once we understand how memory works. Following is an attempt to present, in simple terms, a concise description of the memory process.

How Memory Works

The brain receives information and experiences from the environment in the form of sensory stimuli: visual auditory etc. the received information (stimuli) is registered, encoded, filed/stored and, when required, recalled (retrieved).

In other words, the memory process is a sequence of several mental steps. It is a chain of electrochemical reactions that includes:

Stimuli ==➤ Reception ==➤ Registration ==➤ Encoding ==➤ Storage ==➤ Recall

"Remembering" is the successful retrieval of stored information. When this chain loses one or more of its links, we have memory loss. For example, we forgot the name of that

Harvard professor who was recently introduced to us, because our brain did not register his name when we heard it. Since it was not registered and coded it could not be stored and be there to be recalled. But why was it not registered?

For an experience of information to be registered and coded we have to pay attention to it, to concentrate on it. Or, we have to receive the information repeatedly. We forgot the name of the professor because we did not focus on it when we heard it and besides, we only heard the name once. In contrast, we do recall the name of our elementary school teacher, because we payed attention to it at the time, and also because we heard it multiple times. It was, therefor, registered, encoded, stored and is still available for us to retrieve it. Likewise, we had seen the color of the hair of the professor but we don't remember it, again for the same reason. Antithetically, we do recall the color of the hair of our childhood doll because we had seen it so many times.

Conclusion We will not remember information received at any time if, for whatever reason, it was not registered, encoded and stored; but we will be able to retrieve information and experiences, received even many years ago, if they went through the entire sequence of the memory process and the stored memory has not been decayed over time. To register and encode information we have to pay attention to it, to focus on it and/ or receive it many times.

Short-Term and Long Term Memory and Their Failure

There are two kinds of memory. **Short term**, also referred to as working memory and **Long Term**

The short-term memory is very short. It lasts only seconds, sometimes a few minutes. Long-term memory, on the other hand, can potentially store information for an unlimited period of time.

Long-term memory is stored in the hippocampus, which is a region of the brain near its base. Information from the short-term memory is transferred to the long-term memory.

Loss of long-term memory is due to decay over time or failure of the retrieval process.

Failure of short-term memory is of particular important because, as noted below, it may have potentially serious negative implications. Here are a couple of hypothetical examples to illustrate short-term memory failure:

- We asked somebody for the times. He says *"three twenty-seven"* By the time (seconds) we are ready to adjust our wrist-watch we forgot what time he told us.

Or

- We got a street address over the phone *"285 West 27 Street"* When we attempt to write down, a few seconds after we hang up, we discover that we have already forgotten it.

I cannot resist the temptation of citing an anecdote that illustrates very effectively loss of short term-memory.

> A patient complains to his physician: *"Doctor I have a big problem. I am very concerned. I am losing my memory. This morning, for example, I asked my wife*

what day it is. She said Thursday and within a few seconds I forgot what day she told me. Doctor it is a big problem." The doctor asks: *"How long do you have this problem?"* and the patient says: *"What problem?"*

As stated earlier, short-term memory loss is important because it could have serious implications and might even be dangerous. It may impact our ability to take care of ourselves. It could make driving very risky. Even taking medicine could be unsafe if we do not remember whether we took a pill or which pill we took. Short –term memory failure is also important because it may reflect underlying serious brain disorders. It could, for example, be one of the early signs of Alzheimer's disease.

But we should not get alarmed. In most cases short memory loss is not serious or ominous. The same is true for the long-term memory loss. Occasional, transient, or insignificant lapses of memory, occurring usually in late life, should not be worrisome. Aging is not necessarily entwined with dramatic memory loss. The forgetfulness of older people is normal. It is, one could say, a "normal abnormality".

Normal memory failures are not disabling. They are not affecting our ability to function and carry out normal activities.

The assessment of the gravity of a memory loss should include questions like:

- Does it disrupt the daily routine?
- What is being forgotten?
- How often do the lapses occur?
- Are there signs of confusion, loss of orientation or other symptoms of cognitive failure?
- Is the memory loss getting worse?

Here are a few examples to make clear the distinction between normal forgetfulness and pathologic, serious memory loss.

- If we forgot the name of the hotel at which we stayed in Athens last summer, it is not a big deal. But not remembering that we went to Athens last summer, raises a red flag.
- If we don't remember the square footage of our summer house it is not a major crime. But not remembering that we have a summer house, rings the alarm bell.
- To forget where parked our car may be frustrating but not something to be concerned about. What is alarming is the failure to remember where we are and how to get home.

To portray the potential risks of this kind of memory loss here is another anecdote which dramatically illustrates a life-threatening possibility.

A young lady calls and warns her grandfather who is driving on the Expressway : *"Grandpa be careful. I heard in the news that someone, probably drunk or crazy, is driving on the Expressway against the traffic."* And the grandfather responds: *"I see him, I see him. But there is more than one. There are many!!*

Conclusion Both, long and short-term memory loss can either be normal forgetfulness, usually occurring in old age, or serious, pathologic memory failure impacting activities of routine daily life.

Risk Factors and Causes of Memory Loss

There are several factors, both intrinsic and extrinsic, that cause memory loss or contribute to its development. They may act singly or in combination. Some of them are manageable, others are beyond our control.

The following list of causes and risk factor will give you a clue of what remedial steps and preventative measures are recommended.

Genetics

Our knowledge of the role of genetics in memory is very limited. Probably multiple genes are involved in the progressive decline of cognitive functions, acting through several mechanisms.

Gender

Statistical studies indicate that cognitive failures are more prevalent in females as is the case for the incidence of Alzheimer's disease.

Aging

As we are getting older our muscles become weaker and our cognitive activities, particularly memory, decline. Failure of memory is due to the fact that in the golden years of our life, parts of our brain involved in memory, particularly the long-term memory depository hippocampus, decay and shrink.

Contributing to those age-related retrogressive changes are: genetic factors, including a reduction of the genes that play a central role in memory[80]; poor cerebral blood circulation; and reduced levels of proteins and other agents that stimulate neurogenesis (growth of new nerve cells and formation of new synapses)

Smoking

The nicotine and other toxic substances, contained in tobacco smoke, cause constriction of the cranial vessels. This vasoconstriction results in narrowing of the vascular lumen which, in turn, causes a reduction in the blood flow. The ensuing fall in the amount of nutrients and oxygen delivered to the brain leads to atrophy of cerebral tissue.

Alcohol Abuse

Too much alcohol is toxic to neurons (nerve cells). One reason that excessive alcohol consumption harms neurons is the deficiency of vitamin B1 that it causes

Vitamin Deficiency

Deficiency of vitamins B1, B12, E, D.

Dehydration

Medications

Some medications may potentially contribute to memory problems. They include analgesics (pain killers), sedatives, tranquilizers, drugs for depression, for hypertension and others.

Brain Injury

Cranial trauma, brain tumors, stroke

Brain Disorders

Dementia, Alzheimer's Disease

Hypertension, Diabetes Mellitus, Cholesterolemia

Increased blood pressure, sugar, or cholesterol may cause blood-vessel damage leading to a decreased supply of oxygen and nutrients to the brain.

Obesity

Defined as a BMI Index (Body Mass Index) higher than 30. The frequent association of obesity with diabetes and hypertension increases the risk.

Sleep Deprivation

Sleep enhances the ability of the brain to consolidate, store and retain memories by strengthening *synapses* (neural connections) Lack of sleep causes a reduction in the formation of the new nerve cells in the hippocampus.

Stress, Anxiety, Depression

In stressful situations, the adrenals secrete several hormones, including cortisol, to helps the body cope with stress. Cortisol, however, has also some negative effects. It impacts the hippocampus. The longer or more frequent the stress the more severe the damage[81]. Over time, the assault on the hippocampus results in atrophy.

Conclusion There are several factors both, intrinsic and extrinsic that cause memory loss or contribute to its development.

Prevention of Memory Loss

Introduction

It was already stated that old age is not necessarily entwined with serious memory loss. Older individuals should not inevitably experience significant cognitive decline and memory failure. Or, at least, not a memory loss severe enough to impact normal functions, including the ability to carry our intellectual activities. Take me as an example. Entering my 95th year of age I experience no serious memory problems. I give lectures extemporaneously, without a prompter and without notes. And, of course, I am writing this book!

Is it true, however, that in our world of increasing longevity, there is an increasing number of people who suffer memory deterioration. This has stimulated an increased interest in the prevention of cognitive decline and memory loss.

There are several measures we can take that may prevent memory problems. Most of the external causative and risk factors e.g., smoking, vitamin deficiency etc, are avoidable and potentially reversible. Some other factors, on the other hand, are beyond our control.

There is nothing we can do, for instance, at least at present, to control the influence of our genes on memory.

Genetic intervention is an approach for the future. It is also true that our knowledge of the pathogenesis of dementia and Alzheimer's disease, which exhibit dramatic memory loss, is not sufficient to enable development of preventive measures. With most of causative and risk factors, however, the cognitive decline and memory loss can, potentially, be averted, ameliorated, prevented from getting worse and even reversed, as it has been shown by numerous studies conducted in the USA and abroad.

The guidelines and instructions that follow will help many readers avoid memory loss. And those who already developed memory problems, might be able to reverse the failure and improve their memory.

Any one of these instructions has the potential of reducing, to a degree, the possibility of experiencing serious memory problems. The more instructions followed, however, the greater the protective effect. This was demonstrated by several studies, including one by UCLA and by the International Longevity Center, which recommends multiple instructions to keep the mind in good functionality[84]. Also, the American Heart Association and the American Stroke Association advised to follow all of seven recommendations to preserve cognitive function.[85]

My prescription for a better memory is not a magic pill. There are no medicines that can effectively prevent or reverse memory loss.

The recommendations and advice that I offer concern lifestyle. They are selective interventions in the daily routine. For this reason, they will probably be in conflict with habits, preferences and conveniences. It will require motivation, willpower and discipline to implement the necessary changes.

My instructions are divided into two groups. <u>What We Should Do</u> and <u>What We Should Avoid</u>. Some of these instructions are similar to those that were suggested for the preservation of youth in Part 2 of the book.

What We Should Avoid

The following are potential causative or risk factors that can either be avoided or corrected by appropriate treatment.

<u>Smoking</u>

As explained earlier, tobacco smoke causes a reduction in the supply of oxygen and nutrients to the brain resulting in atrophy of nerve tissue and consequent decline of mental functions. There are several methods to quit smoking including patches, hypnosis, medications and, of course, plain simple determination and willpower.

<u>Alcohol</u>

Excessive alcohol consumption, in addition to other harmful effects, causes vitamin B1 deficiency that harms the brain and contributes to memory loss. Ideally drinking should not exceed 1-2 glasses of wine per day. Preferably red wine, because of the antioxidant effect of the flavonoids that red wine contains.

<u>Dehydration</u>

Water constitutes over 60% of our body weight and adequate intake of water is an essential requirement for normal body functions, including having a sound memory. What the daily water intake should be depends on how much water we lose through perspiration, respiration, urination and bowel movement. According to the National Academy of Sciences, Engineering, and Medicine, the daily requirement of fluid (not just water) for men is 3.7 and for women 2.7 liters. Other scientists recommend to aim for 6-8 glasses of water per day. We should consider that we also receive an appreciable amount of water through our food and drinks. All this makes it difficult to determine the precise amount of water required. I would say we should drink plenty of water when thirsty. Special attention to their water requirement should be given, however, to those who seldom get thirsty and by those who suffer from diabetes or some kidney disorders or those who take diuretics, or laxatives.

Vitamin Deficiency

Vitamins, particularly vitamin B1, B12, E and D, play important roles in the memory process. A balance diet containing lots of fruit and vegetable provide adequate amounts of vitamins. People who do not consume sufficient amounts of those important nutrients should receive supplemental medication. Pills or a monthly injection of vitamin B12 may be required for vegetarians, because vitamin B12 can only be found in red meat.

Obesity

Obesity impacts health in several ways. Among other ill effects, obese (BMI over 30) and overweight (BMI 25-30) people have a higher risk, than those with normal weight of developing dementia and memory loss.

Four factors are crucial for the maintenance of normal weight: diet; exercise; willpower; and discipline.

Hypertension, Diabetes Mellitus, Cholinesterolemia

It was already stated that abnormal levels of any of the above conditions may cause damage to blood vessels eventually leading to brain atrophy[82]. All of them are reversible risk factors since all three can be treated. If you suffer from any of those, your physician has, probably, already prescribed appropriate medications and diet.

<u>Stress, Anxiety, Depression</u>

Each of the above three conditions impacts memory. Whenever possible, persisting attempts should be made to resolve or, at least, alleviate the severity of the problems that created those conditions.

Unfortunately, in most cases this will be easy to say but hard to do.

Engaging in social interactions could help ward off stress and depression. Relaxing exercises such as yoga, may also help.

It might be appropriate, at this point, to mention an exercise that could lower the intensity of those conditions. I refer to it as "cyclic respiration". Normal breathing has three phases

Breathe in—Breathe out—Pause...............
Breathe in—Breathe out—Pause..............

In cyclic respiration we skip the pause. Each cycle is immediately followed by the next

Breathe in—Breathe out--Breathe in—Breathe out

This respiration, particularly in combination with relaxing exercises, may provide at least a temporary relief.

<u>Sedentary Life</u>

Prolonged immobility affects negatively the cardiovascular system. This could lead to a reduction in the flow of blood to the brain and possible cerebral atrophy.

It is recommended that after one hour of sitting to take a walk for about three to five minutes.

<u>Certain Medications</u>

Some prescription drugs, e.g. certain antihypertensives, statins, antidepressants etc, may have side effects that impact memory.

Even over-the-counter medications can cause memory problems. Such medications include antihistamines, *analgesics* (pain killers), sedatives, tranquilizers and sleeping pills.

Individuals, particularly seniors, who receive multiple medications have a higher risk of developing memory problems.

In a recent study it was observed that loss of gray matter was more pronounced in the brains of people who were on three or more medications.[83]

Patients on prescription drugs experiencing memory failures should discuss the problem with their physicians who may, if necessary, change prescriptions or make appropriate adjustments.

What We Should Do

Most of these instructions give choices. Selecting the choices that are more pleasurable or convenient will provide greater adherence, consistency and continuity, which are important for the successful mediation of benefits. Before you adopt any particular diet you should consult your physician.

<u>Eat the Right Food</u>

Our diet should contain:

1. <u>Fruits and Vegetables</u>. Lots of them. As it was mentioned in Part 2, Instruction #1 of this book, fruits and vegetables, particularly those with green leaves, contain flavonoids. These are antioxidants that neutralize the oxidative action of free radicals that destroys tissues in the brain.
2. <u>Omega3 Fatty Acids</u>. The brain consists 60% of fat of which 30% is Omega3 fatty acids. Foods rich in Omega3 fatty acids are tuna, salmon, sardines, trout, and walnuts.
3. <u>Oils</u>. We should eat polyunsaturated fats such as olive oil. Avoid saturated and trans fats. No butter and creams and no cheeses and dairy products with high content of fats.
4. <u>Vitamins B, Particularly B1 &B12, E and D</u>. Vitamin B12, protects neurons and is involved in the synthesis of *neurotransmitters* (substances that transmit nerve impulses from one neuron to another). It is present only in red meat and, as stated earlier, people who do not eat red meat probably need supplementation. Vitamin E is an antioxidant and retards neurodegeneration. It is found in eggs, avocado, almonds and walnuts.
5. <u>Adequate Amounts of Protein</u>. Primarily from fish, skinless poultry and from legumes such as beans and lentils.

6. <u>Reasonable Amounts of Calories</u>. Reduce as much as possible the consumption of carbohydrates (starch and sugar) and fats.

Get Plenty of Sleep

Adequate sleep is necessary for the normal function of memory. Sleep strengthens *synapses* (communications between nerve cells), and plays a role in consolidation, moving data from short to long-term memory, and in the storage and retention of memories in the hippocampus. Sleep deprivation causes a reduction in the growth of new neurons in the hippocampus. It is recommended a night-time sleep of 7-8 hours and a nap of 30-60 minutes. Try to establish a sleeping routine, going to bed and getting up at the same time everyday.

Napping, still culturally unacceptable in the USA, is recommended because it enhances cognitive performance and boosts memory.

It also improves alertness and supplements insufficient night-time sleep.

Engage in Intellectual Activities

We should stay intellectually active. Read books, magazines, newspapers, learn a foreign language, a new skill, or learn to play a musical instrument. Play games such as bridge, chess, Scrabble or solve crossword puzzles, and Sudoku. The more enjoyable and stimulating those activities, the greater their energizing effect on the brain.

Engaging the brain in intellectual activities also enriches the so-called Cognitive Reserve, which is the combined protective effect gained from the educational attainments, occupation and cognitive activities during a lifetime. People with high cognitive reserve have a low risk of suffering memory problems.[86]

Low intensity cognitive training programs can also alleviate cognitive deficits and improve memory failures, as could computerized cognitive retraining like Lumosity, CogniFit Brain Fitness and others.[90]

Engage in Social Activities

Get together with friends and relatives. These social interactions enhance memory, particularly when the discussions are about past or upcoming events and future plans. Volunteer for charitable organizations or for the local school. Join a book club. People who are not engage in social interactions have a higher risk of experiencing memory problems. Engaging in social activities is particularly important for people who live alone.

Set Goals and Targets

In a previous chapter (Part 2, Instruction #3) it is stated that dreaming, having goals and setting targets are important elements of our quest for longer youth. They are also important factors for the maintenance of sound memory. The challenges, anticipation and the emotional excitement of dreaming and planning, that goals and targets create, stimulate cognitive functions and improve memory.

The goals and targets, as mentioned earlier, can be important or trivial; short-term or long-term; performance; or learning goals.

Exercise

Physical exercise is the most important activity that potentially can prevent, ameliorate, delay and even reverse memory failures.

To function normally, the brain requires two indispensable provisions: oxygen and nutrients. It is the circulating blood that brings oxygen and nutrients to the brain and it is the pumping action of the heart that circulates the blood and sends it to the brain. Physical exercise improves blood circulation by causing an increase in the rate and strength of the heartbeat. This results in an increased blood flow and improved perfusion of the brain.

Exercise stimulates the brain's ability to make new synapses and to preserve them.

Previously it was believed that the brain cannot generate new brain tissue. This is no longer true. The brain *is* capable of producing new nerve cells and new pathways. Exercise promotes neurogenesis (creation of new nerve cells) and stimulates synthesis of neurotransmitters in the hippocampus[87]. Supporting this beneficiary effect of physical exercise was the finding that the volume of the hippocampus, which shrinks with age, is increased following physical activity.

Recent studies produced more supporting evidence. Scientists at the University of Maryland have shown, using fMRI (functional Magnetic Resonance Imaging) that a 30-minute moderate exercise (stationary bicycle) increased neural activity in the circuits of several regions of the brain including the hippocampus.[88] There is a plethora of studies that demonstrate the unquestionable beneficial effect of physical exercise on memory.

A study on the Global Ageing & Adult Health of the World Health Organization on 32,715 patients showed that patients who followed the 150 minutes per week regime had lesser cognitive impairment, (which includes memory loss), than those patients who did not exercise.

In a report from the American Academy of Neurology, seniors who walked 6-9 miles per week had less brain shrinkage and more gray matter than those who did not walk[83].

Controlled studies demonstrated that 6 months of moderate daily walking could reliably reverse age-related cognitive decline[50].

Cognitive failure reversal by exercise was also recently observed in an extensive research by scientist of the Mayo Clinic.

The numerous scientific research conducted on the subject, leaves no doubt that physical exercise plays a pivotal role in the prevention, improvement and maintenance of sound memory.

Now, how much and what kind of exercise is recommended? We need light to moderate aerobic exercises such as walking, swimming, bicycling, and even dancing. We can also include some muscle strengthening exercises. As to how much exercise we need the prevailing recommendation from several academic institutions, organizations and agencies, is 150 min per week. Even a little less than that will be beneficial. Before you are engaged in any exercise regimen you should consult your physician.

<u>Medications</u>

Unfortunately there are no medications that will permanently and effectively prevent or reverse memory deficits. Most of the drugs that may provide temporary relief, are cholinesterase inhibitors. Nerve impulses are transmitted from one neuron to another, via synapses, by means of neurotransmitters. One such neurotransmitter is acetylcholine. An enzyme, called cholinesterase destroys acetylcholine and impairs nerve impulse transmission. The cholinesterase inhibitors block the action of the enzyme thus preserving the neurotransmitter acetylcholine.

Among FDA-approved drugs in this category are: Exelon, Donepezil, Memantine and others.

Several herbs, plant extracts and other natural remedies have been proposed as treatments for memory problems but none, so far, met expectations. Among them the controversial extract from the leaves of Ginkgo biloba thought by many to be a rising star. Some scientists, however, feel that Ginkgo hasn't lived up to its early promise[89].

Practical Tips

Here are a few tips to help compensate for memory problems.

- Use a large calendar to mark for birthdays, anniversaries, doctor appointments, meetings, deadlines etc. Consult this calendar every morning.
- Have a folder for pending matters. Place in this folder documents such as receipts, bills, correspondence, notices, forms, etc related to pending issues. Review this folder periodically for the possibility that it is time for action or for follow-up.
- Select specific convenient spots where you always, consistently, deposit your keys, or reading glasses, your wallet or your gloves
- Get a compartmentalized box labeled for each day of the week and deposit in each compartment the pills you will need to take the corresponding day. Such labeled boxes are commercially available.
- Every evening make a list of what you have to do the next day

It is hoped that the readers will implement several, if not all, of the above instructions, but in case they will carry out only one, let that one be:

EXERCISE!!!

Conclusion prevention of memory failures requires avoidance of certain risk factors, e.g. smoking, and vitamin deficiency; appropriate diet; sufficient sleep; intellectual and social engagement and, most of all, physical exercise.

Epilogue

While studying the aging process and methods for averting aging-related functional deficits, we should not disregard the fact that our genetic makeup plays a pivotal role. Scientists are currently exploring relevant DNA segments and testing genetic manipulations in an attempt to ameliorate aging.

Likewise we should not underestimate and ignore the profound effect that a positive change in our mind-set may have on the aging process.

My prescriptions require such a positive change in mentality and recommend corresponding behavioral precepts and guidelines that could delay the onset and attenuate the severity of the functional failures that accompany old age.

No miracles are expected, but it is hoped, that if we follow the instructions given, if we exercise regularly, eat the right food and make the required changes in mindset, attitude, and lifestyle, we may live a little younger a little longer and with less memory problems.

References

1   Bowling A and Dieppe P BMJ 2005; 331: 1548
2   Rowe JW and Kann RL Successful Aging New York Pantheon Books 1998
3   Herodotus Book III: 23
4   Mandeville J The Travels of Sir John Mandeville
5   Oviedo GF Historia General y Natural de los Indias book 16 chapter XI6.
6   Douglas PT "Misconceptions and Myths Related to the Fountains of Youth and John Ponce de Leon 1513 Exploration Voyage" (PDF) New World Explorers, Inc.
7   Glick TF et al Medieval Science, Technology and Medicine 2005: p.20
8   Milbury PE and Richer AC "Understanding the Antioxidant Controversy: Scrutinizing the "Fountain of Youth" Praeger 2007
9   The Tang of Tibet Yoga Journal (http://wwwjogjournal.com/Wisdom/464?page=4)
10 Keler P and Siegel S "Ancient Secret of the Fountain of Youth" 1999 Double Day Book 2
11 "The Five Tibetan Rites-The Truth versus the Claims" (http://www.tst.com/article_info.php!articles_id=19)
12 Bliss S (http://guardianLv.com/author/stasiabliss) 2013

13 Macrae F Daily Mail 2010 Nov 29

14 Piper MD Cell Metabolism 2008; 6: 99-104

15 Bartus RT J Am Geriatr Soc 1990; 38: 680-685

16 Joseph JA Neurobiol Aging 1983; 4: 313

17 Harman D Journal of Gerontology 1956; 11(3): 298-300

18 Assmann KE et al Am J Epidemiol 2015; 182(8): 694-704

19 Joseph JA et al Am J Clin Nutr 2005; 81(suppl): 313S-316S

20 Joseph JA et al J Neurosci 1998; 18: 8047-8055

21 Youdim KA and Joseph JA Free Radic Biol Med 2001; 30: 583-594

22 Cao G et al J Agric Food Chem 1996; 44: 3426-3431

23 Rosedale R J Appl Res 2009; 9: 159-165

24 Rosedale R et al J Appl Res 2009; 9: 159-165

25 Mozaffarian D Atheroscler Suppl 2006; 7: 29-32

26 Bengmark S Curr Opin Clin Nutr Metab Care 2006; 9: 2-7

27 Hayes DP Eur J Clin Nutr 2007; 61: 147-159

28 Scorupa DA Aging Cell 2008; 7: 478-490

29 Solon SM Cell Metab 2014; 19: 418-430

30 Lee KP Proc Nat Acad Sci USA 2008; 105: 2498-2503

31 American Council on Science and Health 2003

32 Ortiz A Ont J Dermatol 2012; 51(3): 250-262

33 Gatherwright J et al Plasr Reconstr Surg 2012; 130(6): 1219-1226

34 Lahmann C et al Lancet 2001; 24: 935-936

35 Morita A J Dermatol Sci 2007; 48(3): 169-175

36 Reid RD et al Patient Educ Couns 2009; 76(1): 99-105

37 Grogan S et al Br J Health Psychol 2009; 14(pt1): 175-186

38 Grogan S et al Br J Health Psychol 2011; 16(4): 475-489

39 Lopez EN et al Health Psychol 2008; 27: S243-251

40 "Alcohol and Aging" Alcohol Alert 1998; No 40

41 Spencer RL and Hatchison KE 1999; 23:No 4

42 Moss S et al J Royal Coll Gen Pract 2014; 64(618): 47-53

43 Cochrane Collaboration Cochrane Database of Systematic Reviews 2012; 10: Art No CD 009009

44 Emerson H JAMA 1923; 80: 1376

45 Frame DS and Carlson SJ J Fam Pract 1975; 2(1): 29-36

47 US Preventive Services Task Force. "Guide to Clinical Preventive Services: Report of the Preventive Services Task Force" 2nd Ed Williams & Wilkins 1996

48 Campbells et al J Am Geriatr Soc 2011; 54(2): 224-232

49 Victor Agingsciences 2011; August 2

50 Erickson KI and Kramer AF Br J Sports Med 2009; 43: 22-24

51 Navaro et al Am J Physiology 2004; 264(3)

52 Rogers MA Exercise & Sport Sciences Reviews 1993; 21(1): 65-102

53 Campeau DS et al The Journal of Neuroscience 2011; 31(22): 11578-11586

54 Kim SE et al Experimental Gerontology 2010; 45(5): 357-365

55 Kramer AF Psychological Science 2003; 14(2): 125-130

56 Kaliman P Ageing Research Reviews 2011; 10: 475-486

57 McAuley E and Rudolph D Journal of Aging and Physical Activity 1995; 3: 67-96

58 Buckwalter JA Physician Sport Med 1997; 25: 126-126, 130-133

59 Daley MJ and Spinks WL Sports Med 2000; 29(1): 1-12

60 Judge JO et al Phys Ther 1993; 73: 254-262

61 Buchner DM West J Med 1997; 167: 258-264

62 Hayes WC et al Bone 1996; 18: 77-86S

63 Dustman RE Neurobiology of Aging 1984; 5(1): 35-42

64 Walton AG Forbs 2013; Nov 12

65 Cock E Daily Mail 2015; Dec 4

66 Hughes JR Preventive Medicine 1984; 13(1): 66-78

67 Byrne A and Byrne DG Journal of Psychosomatic Research 1993; 37(6): 565-574

68 Petruzzello SJ Sports Medicine 1991; 11(3): 143-182

69 Rivera V American Fitness Professionals & Associates 2013; April 10

70 Dzewaltowski OA Res & Exerc Sport 1986; 57: 67-169

71 Viamontes GI and Nemeroff CB Psychiatric Annals 2009; 39(12): 973-998

72 Scheiner MF & Carver CS Current Directions in Physiological Science 1993; 2(1): 26-30

73 Levy BR et al J Gerontol Psychol Sci 2002; 57(5): 409-417

74 Kenton L "Healthy and Lean for Life" Feb 4, 2013

75 West R et al "New Developments in Goal Setting and Task Performance" Routledge 2013

76 Mettlin C and Dodd GD CA Cancer J Clin 1991; 41(5): 279-282

77 American College of Physicians Ann Intern Med 1981; 95(6): 729-732

78 Mastroiacovo D et al Am J Clin Nutr 2015; 101: 538-548

79 Baddelay A Working Memory; Thought and Action Oxford University Press 2007

80 Lu T et al Nature 2004; 429:883-91

81 Conrad CD Psychiatry 2010; 34:742-755

82 Nagai M et al Am J Hyperten. 2010; 23:116-124

83 Smith M et al HelpGuide June 2019

84 Int. Longevity Ctr Report on Memory July 2007

85 Diener HC News & Perspective February 2018

86 Marioni R et al The Gerondologist 2009; 49: 61-71

88 Lowry F Medscape June 2019

89 Graff-Radfort J Mayo CI Patient Care & Health Info Oct. 2019

90 Kueider A et al PIoS one 7.7 2012; e40588

The cover was designed by **Depy Chryssanthou**